# ENDORSEMENTS

Dr. Suka explains a scientifically proven cause of addiction and gives us a clear path to sustained recovery through restoring dysfunctional brain chemistry. When we move to greater understanding about the addiction process, anger is replaced with compassion and forgiveness. Lives of individuals and families could be saved from reading this do-it-yourself book.

*Stan Stokes, MS, LPC, CCDC*
*Founder and Director of Bridging the Gaps Treatment Facility*
*Founder of Alliance for Addiction Solutions*


As I read Dr. Suka's book, I kept thinking how far-reaching it could be. How it could change the whole trajectory of the substance abuse treatment industry. As a doctor of clinical psychology and advanced substance abuse counselor, I am convinced an understanding and utilization of the RDS concepts by competent professionals will create higher rates of recovery success, less loss of life, and improved quality of life for our families, our communities, and our country.

*Dr. Lin Hogan, PsyD, LPC, CRAADC*
*Clinical Therapist and Advanced Substance Abuse Counselor*


This book provides truly enlightening information that can help an estimated 18-million people who are suffering from the pain of addictions! Imbalances within the brain chemistry must be corrected and this information needs to become public knowledge. Dr. Suka reveals the underlying cause of addictions and provides the information that can release these millions from the entrapment of addiction.

Addiction recovery truly has nothing to do with "willpower" or "if you would only just stop drinking" attitudes. Addiction recovery does rely on following through with the suggestions in this book in order to get amazing results. So, if you are addicted to alcohol, I implore you to read this book and follow it, or provide it to your loved one who has been living with inner pain while attempting to self-medicate with alcohol or drugs.

*Barbara Reed Stitt, Ph.D.*
*Author of Food & Behavior,*
*International Radio/TV personality,*
*Former President of Natural Ovens Bakery*
*Former Chief Probation Officer, Cuyahoga Falls Municipal Court, Ohio*

# HOW TO
# QUIT DRINKING FOR GOOD
# and FEEL GOOD
# *The NEW Alcoholism Story*

## Suka Chapel-Horst, RN, PhD

Brainworks Publishing

HOW TO QUIT DRINKING FOR GOOD and FEEL GOOD
THE NEW ALCOHOLISM STORY

Author: Suka Chapel-Horst, RN, PhD
www.AriseAlcoholRecovery.com
www.BrainworksAlcoholRecovery.com

Brainworks Publishing
Copyright © 2013 Suka Chapel-Horst, RN, PhD
Library of Congress Cataloging-in-Publication Data
Library of Congress Control Number: 2013940722
Brainworks Publishing
Hendersonville, NC

ISBN-10: 0615817556
ISBN-13: 9780615817552

# DEDICATION

This book is dedicated to all those suffering from the disease of alcoholism, both present and past, including families and loved ones. Your experience has paved the way for a new day of awareness. This book is also dedicated to the neuroscience and biochemical researchers and healthcare professionals who have bravely stepped outside-the-box to create new recovery models using an all natural approach to freedom from addiction.

You are the Wayshowers.

# CONTENTS

# ACKNOWLEDGMENTS

I am indebted to so many that it would be unfair to attempt to mention them all. However, I do want to pay special tribute to Keith W. Sehnert, MD, who encouraged and assisted me on this path, to Weston Price, DDS, whose amazing groundbreaking research nailed it, to William Crook, MD, who went out on a limb, to James Braly, MD, an allergy pioneer whose work I memorized when I founded my first Optimal Health Program in Minneapolis years ago, to Carl Pfeiffer, MD, PhD and Abram Hoffer, MD, pioneers in orthomolecular medicine, and to Charles Gant, MD, who wouldn't be stopped, to Joan Mathews-Larson, PhD, whose pioneering work guided me from the beginning, to Julia Ross, MA, MFT, who is leading us forward, and to Barbara Reed Stitt, PhD, a pioneer who continues to mentor me. To these pioneers, and to the orthomolecular forerunners, starting with Linus Pauling, MD and all the others who have brought us to where we are today, I humbly thank you. I am also indebted to the members of Alliance for Addiction Solutions, an organization that is promoting drug-free brain repair, internationally. Closer to home, I am forever grateful to Ed and Romella Hart-O'Keefe for being the god-parents of *ARISE* Alcohol Recovery™ and Brainworks Alcohol Recovery™ and by holding the vision, supporting and encouraging me, no matter what. And most importantly, I am indebted and grateful to my husband, David Chapel Horst, who encouraged me, offered suggestions, enlarged my vision, and supported me every step of the way. Without him, this book would never have been written.

# FORWARD

In 1989 I was introduced to orthomolecular medicine. At that time I had been nursing for eighteen years in the mental health field, was president of a national educational organization, and a national speaker on topics of personal development.

I had been ordained as a non-denominational minister, with a focus on metaphysics, and had spent a year as an apprentice to a Sioux medicine man. I was a Master Practitioner of Neuro Linguistics and had been trained in many energy healing techniques including Polarity Therapy, Reiki, and others. Still, I felt something was missing.

When I learned about the work of the chemist, Linus Pauling, and orthomolecular medicine, I knew I'd found the answer. I was excited.

As I began to put together a program for weight loss and optimal healing in general, I was introduced to Dr. Keith Sehnert in Minneapolis, Minnesota where I was living. He was the Medical Director for Health Recovery Center, the alcohol recovery program founded and directed by Joan Mathews-Larson, PhD.

Dr. Sehnert introduced me to her paradigm-shifting book, *Seven Weeks to Sobriety,* in which she gave the results of her groundbreaking work with alcohol recovery to the public. Her work profoundly affected and guided me as I developed what became a successful Optimal Health Program for the general public. I was fortunate to have Dr. Keith Sehnert join me as the Medical Director for my program, as well.

The results of that program proved the efficacy of combining micronutrients and healthy nutrition as a way of life. It is not overstated to say that optimal health was restored to hundreds of lives and personal relationships were greatly enhanced as a result of that program. Unfortunately, family needs caused me to close the program and move to another state.

After spending the next fourteen years as a nurse in the addiction field and criminal justice system, I was appalled at the lack of knowledge and lack of interest in finding solutions for the addicted, especially when the answers have been there all along. It was only a matter of time before I would again join those who are making long-term, symptom-free addiction recovery a reality.

In 2009 I created an Intensive Outpatient Program for alcohol recovery which ultimately led to creating Do-It-Yourself early intervention programs using an alternative biochemical approach. In 2013 my husband, a recovery coach, and I opened an individualized residential treatment and aftercare program for highly functioning individuals who have relapsed following traditional treatment programs and support groups, and for those who are seeking a biochemical alternative to 12 step programs.

In addition I give presentations and workshops to educate people about natural biochemical restoration methods for recovery from addictions, mood disorders, and mental illness. Educating the public and health care providers, and assisting individuals to make a full recovery from alcoholism, is my life passion. We are learning more every day about this disease and how to resolve it naturally by treating the underlying cause, however, medical schools fail to pass this information on to their students. That leaves it up to us to get the message and the help to those who will benefit from it.

# INTRODUCTION

This is a bottom-line book, simple, and to the point. I assume (yes, I know what that means) the reader has little time, energy or desire for lengthy research details and background material. I refer you to the resources at the end of the book for more in-depth information.

It's more important to go with your gut. Does this information make sense? Does it resonate with you? To the alcoholic, I ask, *"Are you are motivated and committed to do what it takes to recover for good and feel good?"*

In this book, I will give you a layman's understanding of the neuroscientific cause of addiction and provide a biochemical approach to recovery.

As always, there are individual differences that need to be addressed in the recovery process. The recovery process outlined in this book is designed to guide highly functional individuals to recover before the complications of advanced alcoholism take over.

Furthermore, the information in this book will assist those who are currently recovering from alcoholism (have sobriety) but have been unable to release the symptoms known as Chronic Abstinence Symptoms, (more commonly known as "dry-drunk syndrome").

I advise you to check with your health care provider before beginning this recovery program. This program is educational in nature and is not meant to be a substitute for medical advice. Underlying medical conditions that are beyond the scope of this book must also be addressed.

If you are in the midst of this program and discover the need for medical, psychiatric, or counseling intervention, immediately avail yourself of that help.

That said, if you are a highly functioning individual, or even if you are unsure if you are an alcoholic but are experiencing alcohol-related problems, then consult your health care provider for the go-ahead to recover through this program.

If you are following the guidelines in this book and need more information, or assistance, or have questions that are not answered to your satisfaction, you can request a consultation with me, Dr. Suka. If you find you need more individualized guidance and supervision, you might consider the *ARISE* residential program. (See Appendix A.)

My mission is to inform the public and open-minded health care professionals about the real cause and the reversal of drug addiction, specifically addiction to alcohol. It isn't what you've heard in the past. It isn't about guilt, shame or blame and it's not about moral shortcomings. Alcoholism is an inherited, genetic, neuro-biological disease that can be reversed, the sooner the better.

I look forward to the time when all treatment centers incorporate a biochemical and nutritional approach to recovery into their programs.

"Dr. Suka" Chapel-Horst, RN, PhD
May 2013
Etowah, North Carolina

# PART ONE

## *UNDERLYING CAUSE OF ALCOHOLISM*

# THE OLD ALCOHOLISM STORY

My husband and I were at a baseball game when an acquaintance, Kathy, sat down beside me. At first we loudly shared the excitement of a high-fly to right field with two runners on base. Then she began to ask some questions about the Do-It-Yourself alcohol recovery program I had developed.

Her fifty-two year old son was hospitalized with severe heart and lung problems. His physician had just told him he would die if he didn't stop his forty year old drinking habit immediately. Kathy said her son didn't have the money to go to a treatment facility and he probably wouldn't go anyway. He'd been through four treatment programs already and relapsed every time.

This is a heartbreakingly common scenario. The sad part is that it should never have happened. If people think they might have arthritis or diabetes, for example, they're not ashamed to seek early medical attention. Why would they be ashamed? They want to get help to avoid complications and have the best life they can under the circumstances.

Why, then, should the disease of alcoholism be thought of any differently than diabetes or arthritis? Why is alcoholism something to be ashamed of to the point of denying having it and avoiding early intervention?

Of course alcoholism has always been with us and, unfortunately, most addiction treatment models are still operating out of the early mythology of alcoholism. Even with the latest neuroscientific research pointing to both the cause and a highly successful treatment model, traditional treatment programs continue to operate in the dark ages of alcoholic thinking. Why? Because change is so hard to accept when whole belief systems and organizations are built up around what once seemed so valuable.

For example, the Hudson automobile was launched in 1909. Over time it became the heaviest, sturdiest car with the best gas mileage. As time went on, other auto manufacturers developed lighter cars with better fuel mileage, while Hudson refused to adapt to the growing market trend. A stylish and highly desired auto was overtaken by more advanced technology. After 1957, when the last car rolled off the production line, Hudson became obsolete because it had refused to change.

Even today, Kodak suffered from staying with film while the rest of the industry was going digital. Change is a normal and inescapable part of life. Things and ideas that refuse to change stagnate and eventually become obsolete. Automobile styles change every year. Companies change their product's color, sizes, shapes and prices. Advertising changes to catch our attention. Fashion ideas change. Technology changed from room size computers in the 60's to today's iPods and android cell phones. But, accepted beliefs about alcohol haven't changed since 1935!

When Bill Wilson and Dr. Bob Smith formed Alcoholics Anonymous, they knew nothing about brain chemistry. What they did know was that this disease had been with us since the beginning of recorded time. It was devastating, progressive, and deadly, and at that time, there was no known cure for it.

Dr. Carl Jung in Zurich, Switzerland sent a letter to Bill W. through a mutual friend saying that there was no medical or psychological hope for an alcoholic. The only hope was a spiritual or religious experience or conversion.

In another letter sent to Bill W., he wrote "Marcus Aurelius Antoninus (121-180 A.D.), a great general, philosopher, and Caesar of Rome (161-180 A.D.) wrote in Latin, *Espiritum vinci espiritus* which translates to *Higher Power overcomes alcoholism.*" The letter was signed "From Dr. Carl Gustav Jung," and was dated January 30, 1961.

Bill Wilson was already attending meetings of the evangelical Christian Oxford Group which began as a First Century Christian Fellowship. They espoused the four absolutes: honesty, purity, unselfishness and love. They practiced the principles of self-survey, confession, restitution, and service to others, principles that eventually would lead to the creation of the 12-Steps of AA.

While attending these meetings, Bill had had a religious "conversion experience" that helped him to stop drinking but he still struggled with terrible cravings and other symptoms, and he was frustrated.

In May of 1935 Bill met Dr. Bob Smith, also an Oxford Group member. Dr. Bob was a proctologist and still drinking alcoholic. Bill presented to Dr. Bob the four aspects of his one core idea: alcoholics experience utter hopelessness, they're totally deflated, they require conversion, and they need others. Dr. Bob had a sudden realization that "The spiritual approach was as useless as any other if you soaked it up like a sponge and kept it to yourself." The purpose of life was not to "get"; it was to "give".

Together, Bill and Bob believed that the key to recovery was to reach out to others. They believed that one couldn't recover by oneself. Based upon these beliefs, they founded Alcoholics Anonymous. Bill and Bob remained members of the Oxford Group for two more years. In December of 1938 the 12-steps of AA were written. A careful look at the 12-steps will show how they were influenced by the beliefs and principles of the Oxford Group.

AA has always offered nonjudgmental acceptance, support, understanding and encouragement to alcoholics. True dedication to serving others and genuine love for each other has provided a haven for alcoholics throughout the years when the non-alcoholic world has looked unfavorably upon alcoholics and alcoholism.

When newcomers attend their first AA meeting, they are greeted with immediate warmth, openness, and acceptance. For a long time AA was the only resource for alcoholics and many alcoholics owe their sobriety to AA.

In 1946 AA's 12 Traditions were adopted, forever cementing Alcoholics Anonymous in stone. Not only could AA never change, but it could never have an opinion on outside issues (# 10 of the 12 Traditions.)

The purpose was, of course, to maintain and protect the purpose and principles of AA. What that did, however, was to prevent AA from incorporating any new developments in the field of alcohol research and treatment. And, it stopped Bill Wilson from making the changes he wanted to incorporate into AA in later years. When he tried to recommend nutritional supplements to members of AA, he was told that if he continued to do that, he would have to resign from AA's board of directors.

It is not widely known that Bill Wilson actively investigated the biochemical basis of alcoholism. He had discovered that he was low in Vitamin B-3, Niacin, which we now know is common in alcoholics.

"Wilson met Abram Hoffer [a Canadian biochemist, MD and psychiatrist who was *successfully* treating schizophrenia with nutrition and vitamin therapy]. From Dr. Hoffer, Bill learned about the potential mood-stabilizing effects of niacin. Wilson was impressed with experiments indicating that alcoholics who were given niacin had better sobriety rates, and he began to see niacin 'as completing the third leg in the stool, the physical to complement the spiritual and emotional.'

Wilson also believed that niacin had given him relief from depression, and he promoted the vitamin within the AA community and with the National Institute of Mental Health as a treatment for schizophrenia. However, Wilson created a major furor in AA because he used the AA office and letterhead in his promotion."[1] (See NOTE 1 at end of chapter.)

(According to Wikipedia, common symptoms of Vitamin B-3, a niacin deficiency, include irritability, poor concentration, anxiety, fatigue, restlessness, apathy, depression, decreased tolerance to cold, and diarrhea. Alcoholic patients are typically low in B-3 and experience increased intestinal permeability, leading to negative health outcomes.)

Upon Bill W.'s death, his wife, Lois, wrote a letter about his hopes for continued research in this area. Her letter was published in a pamphlet, *The Vitamin B-3 Therapy: A 3rd Communication to AA's Physicians.* She wrote that her husband, Bill, had become convinced that there was a biochemical connection with alcoholism.

Aldous Huxley, a great admirer of AA, had introduced Bill to two psychiatrists who were researching the biochemistry of alcoholism. Bill was convinced of the truth of their findings and realized he could again help his beloved alcoholics by telling them about the biochemical component of alcoholism.

Bill W. also discovered that the dry-drunk symptoms he was struggling with were due to hypoglycemia (chronic low blood sugar).

Have you noticed how recovering alcoholics gravitate to sugar-laced coffee, sodas, candy, cookies, chips, and doughnuts, as well as to tobacco? Bill was no different. When he removed the sugars from his diet, his recovery stabilized and his dry-drunk symptoms disappeared. Bill's last years were mainly devoted to the spread of this information among alcoholics and other ill persons. He knew that in the early stages of abstinence, many alcoholics simply aren't capable of thinking clearly and are too damaged by alcohol to work the 12-Steps.[2]

There was just one problem. AA was set in stone. Nothing new could be added or changed, even by one of the founders of Alcoholics Anonymous.

AA took a huge step toward becoming obsolete. Like the Hudson automobile, AA has not kept up with the latest neuroscientific research and advanced treatment models.

If Bill Wilson had been able to influence AA, biochemical restoration would now be an accepted and normal part of their recovery program. Unfortunately, this didn't happen. As a result, AA's recovery rate is generally thought to be between 5% to 17%, according to Johnny Allen, a recovering alcoholic and former director of the Johnson Institute, an organization that is committed to finding solutions for addiction problems. Why does AA settle for such a low success rate? Especially when recovering alcoholics are dying from suicide, kidney disease, heart disease, etc. (See NOTE 2 at end of chapter.)

Nevertheless, many recovering alcoholics attribute the fact that they are still alive and sober to AA. Thus, it can be said that when people believe in, and work the AA program, they can become sober. Does that mean they have recovered? That depends.

Sobriety is not the same as recovery. Many recovering alcoholics switch their addiction to AA and make it the center of focus in their lives.

How many sober alcoholics are still suffering from dry-drunk symptoms including insomnia, depression, irritability, anxiety and cravings? This is not recovery. It's clear that something is not working. While acceptance, support and encouragement are undeniably important, they are not enough in most cases. Even at its best, a 17% recovery rate is, in reality, an 83% failure rate. Would we undergo surgery with a heart surgeon who had an 83% failure rate? I think not.

It should be noted that the vast majority of alcoholics either do not or seldom attend AA.[3] Professional people such as attorneys, physicians, nurses, social workers, dentists, and executives, as well as people in law enforcement, are often reluctant to join groups where they will feel exposed and expected to talk about themselves. Rather than go to an AA meeting, they will either go to an expensive treatment program or they will do nothing and continue to drink.

Most alcohol, and other addiction treatment programs in the United States today, are patterned after the Minnesota Model which was developed in the 1940's and adopted in 1959 by the Hazelden Foundation in Center City, Minnesota.

The Minnesota Model is based on the presumption that drinking is a way of dealing with painful emotional or psychological problems, and that once those problems are identified and confronted, the alcoholic will no longer be driven to drink irresponsibly.

It is presumed that the emotional release accompanying group and individual therapy will lower the need for compulsive drinking. The self-knowledge and insights gained about their alcoholic behavior are believed to help alcoholics remain sober after treatment.

The majority of treatment programs in the U.S. use a 12-step approach taken from AA and require attendance at AA meetings several times a week, if not daily. Despite the availability of modern scientific advancements in the field of addiction, this approach continues to be favored by most treatment facilities even though the long-term recovery rate has never risen above 18.2%.[4]

Caring, support, non-judgmental acceptance, understanding, encouragement, self inquiry, forgiveness, and spirituality are necessary components of recovery. When they are incorporated *together* with neuroscientific advances in treatment, the NEW alcoholism story is one of recovery rates up to 85%. Now that is *good* news.


NOTE 1:

Abram Hoffer, MD, PhD, writes candidly of his work and relationship with Bill Wilson in his book, *The Vitamin Cure for Alcoholism.* (Co-authored by Andrew W. Saul, PhD., Published 2009 by Basic Health Publications, Inc.) Read about Bill Wilson's personal healing, research with alcoholics, and disappointed attempts to change AA.


NOTE 2:

In 1990, the Alcoholics Anonymous General Services office (the governing organization overseeing all "autonomous" meetings) published an *internal* memo that was an analysis of a survey period between 1977 and 1989. [Italics mine.]

According to this memo, *"after just one month in the Fellowship, 81% of the new members have already dropped out. After three months, 90% have left, and 95% have discontinued attendance inside one year!"* (Kolenda, 2003, Golden Text Publishing Company) [Italics mine.]

That means that in less than a year, 95% of the people seeking help from AA leave the program. Regardless of the apparent success rate or cost of any 12-step-based treatment program you may be looking at, the 5% success rate of AA after a year eventually becomes the actual program success rate. (97% of residential and intensive outpatient treatment programs use the 12-step approach.)

# THE NEW ALCOHOLISM STORY
# REWARD DEFICIENCY SYNDROME

Eighteen million United States citizens, plus their families and friends, co-workers and employers, clients and customers, are suffering because of the mythology and dark-age misinformation that is still surrounding alcohol addiction. Alcoholics have been made to feel shame, guilt and remorse for having a physical disease that they did not choose.

Misinformed attitudes have caused sufferers of this disease, like outcasts, to hide their drinking, deny their symptoms, and avoid seeking help. Erroneous beliefs still consider alcoholism to be a weakness of will, a character defect, and a moral shortcoming.

Whether people participate in a treatment program, attend AA, or try to quit drinking on their own, *eight out of ten will relapse* in the first six to twelve months of sobriety. This is scandalous. Something is wrong.[1]

### *Why do we continue to do things that don't work?*

Fortunately, there is a successful recovery method that is getting a long term recovery rate of up to 85%. That translates to a better than *eight out of ten recovery rate*. This is the *new* alcoholism story that everyone needs to know. So to begin, what is alcoholism?

## THE ADDICTION LEGACY

Alcoholism is a treatable disease, just like diabetes. When symptoms of alcoholism develop, it should be normal to seek early intervention, get proper treatment, and avoid relapse. No shame, blame or guilt. Why?

In August of 2011 the American Society of Addiction Medicine (ASAM) published their new definition of addictions. In fact, they finally, and officially, announced what many of us have known for over sixty years; that all addictions are the result of imbalanced brain chemistry.

Addictions Reclassified As Brain Disorders
August 15, 2011

The American Society of Addiction Medicine (ASAM) has changed its definition of addiction to focus on the root cause of the addiction: "A *primary*, chronic disease of brain reward, motivation, memory and related *circuitry*." This moves the traditional definition from one based on behavior and process to one *based on brain function.*

"Addictions are not a result of bad behavior; they are a craving that comes directly from an *imbalanced brain* that is seeking the substance or action to balance itself out," states Lee Gerdes, founder and CEO of Brain State Technologies.

"The behavioral problem is a result of brain dysfunction. The pathology in the brain persists for years after you have stopped taking the drug," according to Dr. Nora Volkow, Director of the National Institute of Drug Abuse (NIDA). *(Italics are mine.)*

Alcoholism is caused by a deficiency in brain chemistry. If a person with this deficiency begins drinking, a dependency on alcohol develops in the primitive part of the brain which is *completely* out of conscious control. Alcoholism is a physiological disease, not a personality or mental disorder. And, this may surprise you, the *most* successful method of treatment is all natural and does *not* use medications.

So now, let's get more specific about the cause of alcoholism, and addictions in general.

## ALCOHOLISM - A PRIMARY DISEASE

A primary disease means that it is not caused by something else. It's not caused by depression or a mental disorder. Alcoholism is not caused by ADD or ADHD. It's not caused by poor parenting or a poor environment. It's not caused by stress, divorce, financial problems, job loss, social pressure or any outside factor. No one can become an alcoholic as a result of any of these conditions. Life circumstances or childhood traumas can severely affect one's life, but they cannot cause alcoholism.

How do we know this? Through multiple twin studies and neuroscience research, conducted over a period of thirty years, we now know what causes alcoholism and other addictions. In 1990, the neuroscientist, Kenneth Blum, and his co-scientists, announced the discovery of the gene responsible for addictions in the Journal of American Medical Association and in 1995 Blum named the resulting disorder Reward Deficiency Syndrome, or RDS for short. These scientists had uncovered the underlying cause of all addictions.

RDS is a neurological dysfunction of brain chemistry, usually caused by an inherited, genetic flaw in the DNA. People who are born with RDS, Reward Deficiency Syndrome, will become alcoholic if they start drinking alcohol. They can't avoid it. Alcohol alters brain chemistry in such a way that the craving for alcohol cannot be ignored.

Let me put this in a more personal way. If you inherited RDS, you will become alcoholic if you drink alcohol. If you inherited RDS and you don't drink, you will not become alcoholic. And, if you were not born with RDS, and did not develop it later in life (see *acquired* RDS), you may abuse alcohol, but you will not become an alcoholic no matter how much or how often you drink. (Of course, a long history of alcohol *abuse* can cause psychosocial and medical complications as well.)

People with primary RDS can't continue to drink, even small amounts, without developing a tolerance that requires more and more alcohol to satisfy. It's a physiological response, not an emotional or mental response. If a person can "just quit" drinking, they don't have RDS. They were alcohol *abusers*. They may go to treatment or AA, recover quickly, and believe that everyone can "just quit" like they did. That is unfair because they didn't have RDS to begin with.

People have said to me, while holding a beer or drinking a glass of wine, "I used to be a functional alcoholic. Now I just drink once in awhile. It doesn't bother me a bit." It is highly doubtful that they were actually *addicted* alcoholics. People can abuse alcohol for years and even have severe physical and socioeconomic difficulties because of it, but if they have inherited or acquired RDS, they can't "just quit" drinking.

RDS is not the same for everyone. One person may have more of a neurotransmitter deficiency than another. For someone with a lower deficiency, recovery may be easier than for one with a higher degree of deficiency. This explains why some people can recover from alcoholism easier than others. No two people are alike. Judgment and blame for failure to recover without addressing the underlying cause is based on ignorance and is lacking in compassion.

> *An alcohol abuser has a DESIRE to drink.*
> *An alcoholic NEEDS to drink.*
> *It's not in the mind. It's in the brain chemistry.*

Not all children born into families with a history of addictions will inherit RDS. Although some children with RDS have EEG, or brain wave abnormalities, not all do, so testing is unreliable. RDS can be inherited even if the disorder skips a generation. The safest way to avoid developing alcoholism is to avoid alcohol if there is any history of alcoholism, other addictions, emotional disorders, or mental illness in the family.

## REWARD DEFICIENCY SYNDROME—AN ACQUIRED DISEASE

Not all RDS is inherited. RDS can be *acquired* in response to allergies, molds, heavy metals, toxic chemicals, hormonal changes, disease, malnutrition, prolonged stress, excessive alcohol or drug *abuse,* and the over-prescribing of addictive medications.

For example, we now know that hormonal imbalances in middle-aged women can lead to the development of RDS and addiction.

Some neurotransmitters are produced in the gut and when the gut is compromised the imbalance can lead to RDS which can then lead to addictions.

All too often, people who are suffering from injuries or have post-operative surgical pain are given pain medications that are addictive. Without alternative treatment for pain management, many continue to take their pain medications and become addicted. This is an example of *acquired* RDS.

Depression is the result of a reward deficiency that is sometimes primary and sometimes acquired. When SSRI antidepressants are given, they actually *increase* the reward deficiency over time leading to addiction problems.

Once *acquired* RDS develops, the response by the body is the same as with *primary* RDS.

## SO, HOW DOES IT WORK?

We've learned that *primary* RDS is an inherited disease. Well, how is it inherited? It's encoded in the genetic makeup of each person. Genes are inherited chemical recipes that come from the parents. Half come from the father and half from the mother. Recipes encoded in the DNA determine how much of each protein is needed, as well as when and where and under what circumstances they're needed. These proteins determine everything from eye and hair color to moods and sleep patterns. These genes provide the recipes for neurotransmitter levels in the brain and this is where RDS comes in.

In fact, there are 10 *different* locations on the human genome that code for a predisposition to alcoholism. So there are several different *types* of alcoholics but all are deficient in the amount of proteins, or amino acids, that are necessary to create sufficient amounts of neurotransmitters.

## THE BRAIN'S MESSENGERS

The nervous system carries energy throughout the brain and spinal cord sending messages to every part of the body. Some nerves serve automatic functions such as breathing, heart action, and digestion, while other nerves serve the conscious part of the brain which we can control. Nerves are not a continuous string. They're made up of independent cells that both receive and send messages on to the next nerve cell through electrical impulses.

The messages, or electrical impulses, are carried from one neuron to another by chemical messengers called neurotransmitters. Neurotransmitters are proteins which are made up of amino acids. And, it's the inherited genetic code that determines the protein recipe, how much is produced and how often.

People with *primary* RDS have a different genetic recipe than people with normal levels of neurotransmitters. This genetic recipe, or code, creates a deficiency in one or more of the neurotransmitters. It also reduces the ability of the nerve cells, or neurons, to receive messages by having fewer receptor sites and, as the disease progresses, by closing down some of the existing receptor sites. (*Acquired* RDS, although not genetically caused, works in the same way.)

To keep this simple, of the more than 200 neurotransmitters in the brain, in the case of addictions, we'll consider four main neurotransmitters and their actions on the brain.

- The neurotransmitter (NT) **dopamine** stimulates or excites us. It's called the "feel good" chemical. It governs our abilities to pay attention and to experience excitement and pleasure. I call it the **Energizer Bunny**.
- The neurotransmitter (NT) **serotonin,** or **Sunshine NT,**. is the brain's natural antidepressant. It exerts a soothing influence on unpleasant emotions. It affects moods, sleep, appetite, and perception. ( Julia Ross of Recovery Systems Clinic near San Francisco believes a serotonin deficiency may be affecting more than 80% of Americans. Eric Braverman, MD, believes that only 17% of the population produces enough of this "sunshine" neurotransmitter.)
- The neurotransmitter (NT) **GABA** (gamma amino butyric acid) acts as a sedative and helps to manage stress by alleviating anxiety and worry. It's the **Chill Out NT**.
- The **endorphins** are the brain's natural pain killers. People who are naturally deficient in endorphins don't have the chemical ability to tolerate pain like other people do. They're not wimps. They just don't have the chemistry to handle pain well. Endorphins can also stimulate the release of dopamine and the accompanying "euphoria" or "good feeling". Endorphins are the **Love Bug** (NT) because they make us feel comfortable and loved.

## UN-NATURAL STRESS

In addition to these neurotransmitters, there is a family of molecules (also made of amino acids) that act *like* a neurotransmitter. This group of molecules is called **Corticotropin Releasing Hormone** or **CRH**. It manages the body's response to stress and anxiety by affecting temperature, blood vessel constriction, growth, and metabolism. This system is damaged in almost everyone with the disease of alcoholism with the result that people who are predisposed to alcoholism don't handle stress well. This is not a case of saying to someone, "just chill out." They would if they could, but their brain chemistry is different and "chillin" is difficult.

If a person doesn't handle stress well, isn't it natural that a substance that would help them to be calmer would be useful and welcomed? Alcohol and other drugs become a rewarding way to self-medicate.

## REWARD DEFICIENT

The right amount and combination of neurotransmitters will lead to a sense of well-being (normal sleep patterns, normal pain tolerance, normal anxiety levels). But people with a genetically caused *deficiency* in neurotransmitters experience a sense of incompleteness, an uneasiness, if you will, and increased anxiety. They may be less stress tolerant or have a decreased tolerance for pain.

Almost all alcoholics will tell you that they always felt different from other people. They were more depressed or uneasy, more anxious or uncomfortable, or they may have reacted more to pain than others. There is a saying in AA that *"alcoholics have a hole in their soul that the wind blows through"*. They just never seemed to feel as comfortable or as good as their friends. This is an important piece of information for non-alcoholics to understand and remember. It calls for compassion, not blame.

Now, if the inherited DNA recipe creates a deficiency in one or more of the neurotransmitters, then a "reward deficiency syndrome" results. (A syndrome simply means a grouping of symptoms.) People *with* the deficiency don't experience the same *internal* rewards, or good feelings, that other people do. They're "reward deficient".

For example, people usually get good feelings when they see a cute baby or a beautiful moonrise, or eat a fine dinner, listen to music, experience sex or laughter, or cuddle with a pet. The person with RDS won't have those same warm fuzzy feelings. They don't get a *natural* high.

# EXAMPLES OF REWARD DEFICIENCIES

## DOPAMINE DEFICIENCY SYMPTOMS

| | |
|---|---|
| Depression | Poor memory recall |
| Irritability | Difficulty waking up in the morning |
| Low energy | Laziness |
| Low motivation | Lack of remorse |
| Weight gain | Detachment |
| Sleep disturbances | Social withdrawal |
| Distractibility | Suicidal thoughts |
| Poor concentration | |

## SEROTONIN DEFICIENCY SYMPTOMS

| | |
|---|---|
| Depression | Lack of self confidence |
| Anxiety | Poor concentration |
| Panic attacks | Eating disorders |
| Irrational emotions | Premenstrual Syndrome |
| Anger | Inflexibility |
| Impatience | Decreased sex drive |
| Phobias | Guilt |
| Negativity | Violence |
| Low energy | Antisocial behavior |
| Lack of self esteem | Suicidal thoughts |

## GABA DEFICIENCY SYMPTOMS

| | |
|---|---|
| Anxious | Sleeplessness |
| Nervous | Overwhelmed |
| Panic Attacks | Pressured |
| Exhausted | Overreacting |
| Tense | Seizures |

# ENDORPHIN DEFICIENCY SYMPTOMS

Difficulty experiencing pleasure

Depressed

Low pain tolerance

Chronic pain (e.g. back aches, headaches)

Very emotionally sensitive

Cry easily (e.g. from sentimental TV commercials)

Find it hard to get through losses or grieving

Overly responsible or time urgent

All addictions are the result of a reward deficiency, including addictions to drugs, tobacco, food, porn, gambling, shopping, exercise, internet games, and even addictions to extreme sports.

Addictions, initially, are unconscious physiological attempts to self-medicate or to create the euphoric high that is naturally missing from the brain. As the addiction progresses, it becomes an unconscious physiological *requirement* for survival, overriding all conscious attempts to stop the addiction.

## IS IT REALLY A DRUG OF CHOICE?

Addicted people don't *choose* their addictions. Their genetic coding points to the substance that will provide the missing ingredient.

85-90% of the US population is exposed to alcohol or drugs during their lifetime, so people who are genetically predisposed to addiction are very likely to find the drug that replaces or "fixes" their "reward deficiency". It makes them feel good.

They may experience euphoria for the first time, or relief from depression or anxiety. They may sleep better. Their physical pain may decrease. They're less stressed. In the early stages of addiction, they've found their fix, or reward, and it feels good. So they continue to self medicate without realizing that their fix is sooner or later going to become an addiction and then a means of survival over which they will have no conscious control.

Drugs of abuse mimic natural brain chemistry, but with much greater intensity. So, if a neurotransmitter is deficient, people will be drawn to the drug that provides the missing reward for that specific neurotransmitter.

Teenagers may begin drinking for social reasons, to belong, or to be cool, or they may find relief from allergies, environmental toxins, ADD, or chronic depression. If they have primary or acquired RDS, they will find the drug that makes them feel better and eventually become addicted.

(The unique problem with teenagers who use or abuse substances is that they fail to learn social skills during the critical years when the brain is still developing. Substance abuse inhibits the development of the frontal lobes that control the ability to foresee consequences, control impulses, and make critical decisions affecting behavior.)

So let's take a look at why people are drawn to their specific drug. Remember, these drugs are providing something that is missing in their chemical makeup, and the drugs are making them feel more "normal". ("Normal" includes being able to naturally have euphoric feelings, or less depression, or decreased pain, or less anxiety, providing the "reward" they are looking for.) Note the correlation between the Deficiency, the Substance, and the Result.

# DOPAMINE DEFICIENCY

## SUBSTANCES USED TO PROVIDE THE MISSING REWARD

Cocaine
Crack
Heroin
Amphetamines
Methamphetamine
Ritalin (as addictive as heroin
    and cocaine)

Diet Pills
Caffeine
Sugar (4 times more addictive than cocaine)
Refined Carbohydrates (Junk food)
Tobacco
Marijuana
ALCOHOL

## REWARD

Feel good

Euphoria

# SEROTONIN DEFICIENCY

## SUBSTANCES USED TO PROVIDE THE MISSING REWARD

Wellbutrin
Prozac
Zoloft
Paxil
Tofranil
Trazedone
Effexor
Lexapro

Luvox
Remeron
Serzone
Elavil
Sugar
Refined Carbohydrates (Junk food)
Marijuana
ALCOHOL

## REWARD

Emotional relaxer

Antidepressant

# GABA DEFICIENCY

## SUBSTANCES USED TO PROVIDE THE MISSING REWARD

Benzodiazepines:
    Valium  (Used to be called
    Librium  tranquilizers, now called
    Ativan  "hypnotics" and
    Xanax  "depressants")
    Serax
    Klonipin
Barbiturates:
    Fioricet for migraines

Soma (relaxes brain, not muscles)
Sleep Aids:
    Ambien
    Lunestra
    Restoril
    Prosom
Tobacco
Marijuana
ALCOHOL

# REWARD

Mental relaxer                    Decreases anxiety

# ENDORPHIN DEFICIENCY

## SUBSTANCES USED TO PROVIDE THE MISSING REWARD

| | |
|---|---|
| Heroin | Codeine |
| Morphine | Lortabs |
| Dilaudid | Fentanyl |
| Pallidone | Darvocet |
| Demoral | Avinza |
| Oxycodone | Methadone  (synthetic opiate) |
| Oxycontin | Suboxone  (synthetic opiate) |
| Hydrocodone | Marijuana |
| Vicodin | ALCOHOL |

# REWARD

Reduce pain                    Comfort


The special problem with endorphin-deficient people who have become addicted is that they often have very real pain. They may have back injuries, or joint problems for which the opiate medications were originally prescribed. Opiates are frequently prescribed following surgery. In many cases, the prescriptions just keep coming with little follow-up by the physician.

People become addicted to the opiates for pain relief without having the help of pain management specialists or without insurance coverage for alternative healing modalities. So, recovering from an opiate addiction, without restoring endorphin levels to near normal doesn't resolve the need for pain management. Many people return to their opiates for pain relief.

People become addicted to the opiates for pain relief without having the help of pain management specialists or without insurance coverage for alternative healing modalities. So, recovering from an opiate addiction, without restoring endorphin levels to near normal, doesn't resolve the need for pain management. Many people return to their opiates for pain relief.


## ALCOHOLISM

You probably noticed that alcohol (and marijuana) is listed under all four categories. That's because alcoholics are *deficient in all four neurotransmitters*. Alcoholics need *more* stimulation than other people just to feel good. They need stimulation to decrease anxiety, sleep better, relax, calm their emotions and decrease pain.

## THE PRIMITIVE BRAIN AND RDS

Now, let's understand just what is going on in the brain and how RDS actually works. The top portion of the brain, the neo-cortex, is where activities including reasoning, learning, ability to foresee consequences, impulse control, sensory perception, and emotional responses take place. It's under conscious control.

Underlying the neo-cortex is the old, or primitive brain, the same brain that's in all mammals. One portion of the primitive brain is called the limbic system. It's responsible for survival, fight or flight, reproduction, and hunger. It's a response system to heat, breathing, and danger. Here's the main point to remember. This primitive brain is not under conscious thinking control.

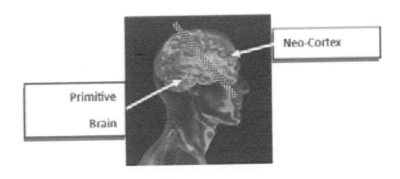

*The REWARD PATHWAY*
*is located in the PRIMITIVE brain.*

*There is NO COMMUNICATION between the*
*Neo-Cortex (thinking) brain and the Primitive Brain.*

Just think of the ramifications of this information. It's useless to attempt to reason with a part of the brain that has no reasoning capability. It's cruel to blame a person or the automatic reactions of a physiological system that is always in survival mode.

Alcoholism and other addictions are a primitive-brain disease. In fact, intelligent people have more difficulty attempting to recover from addictions because they're overconfident. They think they can use their mind to control their addiction, but you can't outsmart the old brain. Motivation and smarts don't matter.

The primitive brain will always trump the thinking or conscious brain when survival is threatened. For example, we know that we can't breathe underwater and survive. If we get water in our lungs, we'll die. Yet, people who have drowned have water in their lungs. So, why did they breathe if they knew that they would die as a result of breathing?

The primitive brain "knows" what is necessary for survival. It "knows" that it must have oxygen to survive. When the oxygen level gets to a certain low point, the brain will make a person breathe no matter how much the conscious mind is telling itself not to breathe.

Drug addiction is like needing oxygen to survive. The primitive brain becomes addicted to the drug and will insist on having it in order to survive. It will cause cravings that are intense gut feelings that *cannot* be ignored. Non-alcoholics don't experience these compelling cravings. What's really going on?

## STEVE'S STORY

Steve has an inherited, genetic deficiency in dopamine, as well as deficiencies in the other neurotransmitters. When he drinks alcohol, the level of dopamine rises in his brain. In the early stages of drinking he feels good, more alive, more alert, and happier than he's ever felt before.

As Steve's drinking increases, over time, the alcohol causes the level of dopamine in his brain to become too high for survival. If the dopamine level were to progress without interference, Steve would develop malignant hyperthermia. His temperature would rise to 110—113 degrees, and he would not be able to survive at that temperature. So the old brain responds to save Steve's life by decreasing the brain's *already reduced* production of dopamine (genetically coded) and by closing down some of the nerve cell's receptor sites so that less dopamine is accepted into the neurons.

Now Steve needs even *more* alcohol to get the *same* dopamine effect. For awhile it goes unnoticed that more and more alcohol is needed to get the fix or reward. Eventually, it becomes obvious that as less and less dopamine is being *naturally* produced by the brain and as more receptor sites shut down, Steve needs more and more alcohol just to feel what he felt before the drinking began. He no longer gets the lift he got when he began drinking. Steve has developed a tolerance to alcohol.

The old brain is in survival mode attempting to keep Steve alive. It must have dopamine and it needs more than it can produce. Steve experiences it as an intense gut-wrenching craving for alcohol. It's *not an emotional desire* to drink or a mental *wanting* a drink. It's a *need* to drink in the same way that the lungs of a drowning person need oxygen to survive and will cause the drowning person to breathe under water.

Steve has *no choice*. He *must* drink to get the dopamine he needs in order to survive, except that drinking no longer provides a sufficient amount to satisfy the primitive brain's requirement for survival, so he is constantly seeking more and more alcohol out of necessity. Can you understand that this is a biochemical disease, not a mental or emotional character defect?

Misinformed people say, *"Steve is drinking too much. He's ruining his life and his health. Can't he see what he's doing and just stop drinking?"* No. He can't just stop drinking. Not only has his thinking brain become impaired by the continued use of alcohol, his thinking brain has no control over the primitive brain which is simply doing what it needs to do to survive.

This is when someone will drink alcohol by the case, or more, on a daily basis, drink mouthwash, drink rubbing alcohol, anything to survive, will steal to get the drug, will prostitute, even commit murder.

Steve has long-ago lost his job, his family, and his possessions, yet he continues to drink. Steve's body is giving up. He has liver disease, diabetes, digestive problems and heartburn, heart and lung problems, yet he's still drinking. Steve is feeling deeply ashamed, scared, hopeless and suicidal, and he's still drinking.

This disease is neither rational nor conscious. It's a biochemical deficiency that is in survival mode. Regardless of all the outer circumstances in Steve's life, his brain needs more dopamine or it will die. So Steve does whatever he has to do in order to get that life-saving, dopamine stimulating, alcohol. And then he drinks it.

Alcohol is *killing* Steve, yet Steve's brain *needs* alcohol-induced dopamine to survive.

## RELAPSE AND DRY-DRUNK SYNDROME

(Now renamed *"Chronic Abstinence Symptoms"*)

Hopefully, long before people get to Steve's depth of alcoholism, they will seek help, and many do. Now the issue becomes, *"Will the help being sought reverse this disease"?* If optimum neurotransmitter levels are not restored, craving and relapse will continue, or at the very least, dry-drunk behaviors will continue, because dysfunctional brain chemistry in the primitive brain remains in survival mode.

### *Relapse is a survival mechanism of the primitive brain.*

Talk therapy and 12 step work do *nothing* to restore neurotransmitter levels. That's why many recovering alcoholics continue to experience poor sleep, anxiety, cravings, irritability, over-reaction to stress, depression, lack of motivation, and a host of other symptoms. And at least 82% to 95% of alcoholics relapse over and over.

The result of repeated relapses is more guilt, more shame and more loss of self esteem. People blame themselves, believing that they lost control. This is the sad story of misinformation. They didn't lose control. Their brain caused them to drink to survive, because they didn't have the proper treatment in the first place.

## CROSS ADDICTIONS

All neurotransmitters affect dopamine release. So cross addictions are common. Many people give up alcohol and then switch addictions to another substance or behavior. Beware. If brain chemistry is not restored to normal, most people will relapse or simply change addictions. Some "recovering" alcoholics think their "marijuana therapy" is harmless.

The new addiction may be to different drugs, or it can be to caffeine, sugar, food, sex, gambling, relationships, or even to AA, for example. All addictions elevate Dopamine levels, including addiction to tobacco.

Eventually, if the damaged brain chemistry is not repaired, people will usually return to their primary addiction. As we will read later, maintaining a tobacco addiction will almost always lead to relapse. And only about 5% of alcoholics can quit on their own (most likely, they had little or low levels of RDS, or were alcohol *abusers*). Those are not good enough odds to take a chance on for one's recovery.

## STARVING TO DEATH

Alcoholism leads to nutritional disaster. Alcoholic individuals are malnourished because they don't eat well, and because their bodies don't metabolize food properly. They're missing the necessary vitamins and minerals that are necessary for rebuilding brain chemistry. (See Chapter 22.)

## THE DOMINO EFFECT

The neo-cortex, or conscious brain, can be severely affected as a *result* of neurotransmitter deficiencies and addiction. Emotional and mental changes occur due to very real changes in the brain chemistry and structures. (See Chapter 29.)

People's lives are negatively affected. Relationships may deteriorate, careers may dry up, finances may plummet, and/or families may be destroyed.

These issues require counseling, therapy, support groups and/or belief management training but only *after* brain chemistry is in recovery mode. Before that, concentration, clear thinking, memory, and emotional stabilization haven't reached a level yet where therapy has much effect.

Most people report that after their brain chemistry is on the mend, their personal life and relationships just naturally seem to improve along with the physiological changes. Issues that were major problems before their brain-repair are not quite so challenging or difficult as they seemed to be in the past.

Remember, the real *cause* of alcoholism, and other addictions, is *not* due to conscious emotional responses or mental choices. Shame, blame, and guilt are absolutely out of place. These responses exist due to ignorance about the real cause of addictions.

## PRE AND CO-EXISTING CONDITIONS

If people have a pre-existing mental illness, also biochemically caused, it will be exacerbated by the substance they are addicted to. Both conditions, the mental illness and the addiction, need to be addressed during and following the addiction recovery process. Any underlying pain or medical condition must be addressed, as well.

## RESCUE

The good news is that when the disease of addiction is treated before medical complications become too severe, the dysfunctional brain chemistry can be restored to normal.

Because the brain chemistry of most people with RDS was deficient from birth, a reversal of that chemistry will release them from a life-long burden and open them to heretofore unknown fulfilling experiences, opportunities, and blessings.

As the physiological *need* for alcohol is erased, recovering alcoholics experience a quality of life that may be the best they have ever felt. The recovering alcoholic will have to deal with the *habit* of drinking in familial, social, and career settings. This needs to be addressed during the recovery phase.

People with severe medical complications from alcoholism will benefit from restoration of brain chemistry, as well. No one should be denied their right to quality of care, especially when bio-restoration of brain chemistry is scientifically and experientially proven and available. What is necessary is for the medical and addiction community to be willing to abandon recovery methods that don't work and adopt proven methods that do work.

So, what's the solution? It's pretty simple, actually. Rebuild the neurotransmitters. Restore the missing elements through biochemical repair and a nutritional program designed to restore the brain and body back to normal. The brain has the ability to repair itself. If you recall, neurotransmitters are proteins, amino acids. Feeding the brain with specific amino acid formulas and other missing nutrients restores brain chemistry to normal.

## NOW, THE BIG QUESTION

If what I've been saying is true, why doesn't everyone know about it, and why aren't the majority of treatment programs using a biochemical approach to recovery? The answer is that many dedicated physicians do know about the real cause of addictions but they haven't been educated in the biochemical approach to recovery. Medical schools don't require either nutritional therapy or addiction education in their programs. If the medical community doesn't know about it, they can't use it. Pharmaceutical companies are embedded with the medical community and have no interest in recovery methods that don't produce profits. Natural nutritional substances, required for full recovery, are not patentable and therefore are not promoted.

It can take a long time for new ideas to become accepted. Ignaz Semmelweis, MD, (1818-1865) is known as the Father of Infection Control. He received a tremendous amount of criticism by his medical peers over his belief that childbed fever was a contagious disease that was spread by the contaminated hands of physicians. (Childbed fever was a common cause of mortality of young mothers.)

Semmelweis was fired from his position as the director of a maternity hospital for suggesting that physicians should wash their hands between patient examinations. Even though mortality rates declined dramatically after medical students began disinfecting their hands with chlorinated lime water, his teachings were not widely accepted among the medical community until long after his death.

Hopefully, as individuals learn about both the cause and cure for addictions, they will demand that rehabilitation facilities provide effective treatment.

## HOLISTIC RECOVERY

While necessary for long-term recovery, the biochemical approach does not stand alone. It must work in combination with other effective tools for body repair, energy balancing, emotional, mental and spiritual recovery. You'll learn more about these in later chapters.

The initial detoxification and recovery process, using a biochemical approach, takes approximately six weeks to ninety days followed by another twelve to twenty-four months, or more, for brain chemistry to be completely restored, depending upon the severity of the addiction. This method of recovery normalizes brain chemistry naturally, allowing one's emotional, mental, and spiritual aspects to reawaken without the interference of mood or mind altering prescription medications.

So now you know the real cause of alcoholism: RDS, Reward Deficiency Syndrome. And you know something about restoring dysfunctional brain chemistry to normal.

For those highly functioning individuals whose alcohol addiction has *not* progressed to medical complications, the Do-It-Yourself Recovery Program outlined in this book may be the answer. (For information on a residential program see Appendix A.)

# FIVE PROFILES 3

Not all alcoholics are the same. Recovery from alcohol requires identifying and treating the underlying bio-chemical imbalances. Specialized micronutrient formulas, vitamin and mineral co-factors, and proper nutrition, coupled with education, will ensure that each person can recover without unexpected relapse.

The following are not real people. The examples are illustrative only.

BRAD has a liver enzyme (alcohol dehydrogenase enzyme) that metabolizes large amounts of alcohol without any negative effects. He doesn't get hangovers. Instead, alcohol stimulates him, gives him more energy and actually improves his performance.

He's usually a Type A personality, always on the go, a high achiever with a high sex drive. He drinks during lunch, has several drinks before dinner, drinks wine with dinner and fills out the evening with one or more after dinner drinks. On weekends, he starts drinking in the early afternoon or late morning. Alcohol never seems to affect him. He can drink most of his friends under the table. He's an intelligent, clever and thoroughly enjoyable person to be around.

Brad's brain makes an endorphin-like substance (tetrahydroisoquinolines) from alcohol which is responsible for both his euphoria and his eventual addiction. Brad doesn't believe he's an alcoholic because he has had a successful career and his work and family life didn't suffer during his early years of drinking. Because the symptoms of alco-holism came on so slowly, he never realized he was hooked on alcohol.

Alas, after fifteen years of heavy drinking, Brad's brain no longer gets the lift and energy it used to get. He needs alcohol just to make it through the day. His former high level of functioning has decreased. His memory and concentration are poor. His liver is becoming diseased.

Now Brad gets severe withdrawal symptoms if he misses his drinks. He has wide emotional swings and fre-quent blackouts. He blames others for his problems. His work, family and personal relationships are suffering. Because of his unique biochemistry, he is classified as an II ADH/THIQ alcoholic.

Brad has primary inherited RDS. He is typical of the majority of alcoholics although their stories differ. Being able to "handle the liquor", "keep up with the boys", and drink large amounts of alcohol socially without apparent effects leads people to think they are not alcoholic. The truth is, it is NOT normal to drink heavily without side effects or getting drunk.

BRENDA is married to a caring and loving husband. She has two children of whom she is very proud. She likes being a wife and mother and tries to provide a loving and supportive home life.

It's difficult for Brenda because she has frequent headaches, is often irritable and is bothered by racing thoughts. She is highly anxious and sometimes acts irrationally which puts her family on the defense not knowing what Brenda will say or do next. Drinking seems to take the edge off it and soothes her mind. She feels depressed and worries about her failure to be the wife and mother she really wants to be.

Brenda doesn't think anyone knows about the alcohol stashed in the closet, and the drinks she secretly takes when no one is looking. She is looking older than her years. Brenda may go for days without a drink and then binges for a week. She has been drinking more frequently and heavily for the last year. Brenda is allergic to wheat products.

Brenda has acquired RDS. Her dependence on alcohol will cease when she identifies her allergies, removes wheat from her diet, checks for other allergies, checks hormone levels, removes toxins from her body, rebalances her brain deficiencies and eats a healthy nutritional diet.

GLEN owns an auto repair shop. He's exposed to paint and other inhaled chemicals every day. After work he heads to a bar for a few beers. Once he starts drinking, he can't stop.

Easily becoming angry once he starts drinking, he sometimes gets into fights. By the time he gets home, he has become agitated and nasty. He takes this anger out on his family.

The next morning he feels sick. He can't remember how much he drank the night before, or even going to the bar. When he learns how he treated his family or friends he is remorseful but he can't remember his actions.

When he gets to work, he starts to feel better. Everyone at work says Glen is really a nice guy, polite and thoughtful. Glen has been drinking for ten years and is allergic to toxic fumes and inhaled chemicals. He has acquired RDS.

STACY is a graphics artist with a well paid position in a respected publishing company. She has earned awards for her creative and novel art work. Recently she has been losing energy and can't seem to concentrate.

Stacy is craving sugar constantly. She can't seem to stop eating candy bars, sodas, doughnuts, potato chips and cookies. She loves her coffee with lots of cream and sugar.

Of course, she's putting on weight as a result. Even worse, Stacy feels bloated and often has diarrhea. Sometimes she breaks into tears for no reason at all. Stacy is getting feedback from her co-workers about being increasingly irritable and argumentative.

She hasn't said anything but she is losing interest in her work and often wants to stay at home. However, drinking helps her feel more like normal.

When Stacy drinks, she isn't as jittery and can get her work done. She is unaware of how much she's really drinking.

Stacy has been drinking socially for ten years. Her drinking has increased over the years but a few months ago she started drinking more frequently and heavily. Stacy has primary RDS and has developed Candida, a yeast overgrowth in her intestine.

ROGER remembers always feeling depressed as a child. He didn't have the energy to play sports and remained withdrawn from most social events. When he was fourteen he discovered that alcohol made him feel normal. He was able to socialize and have fun. So Roger began to drink with the guys and eventually drinking became second nature.

Now, after twenty years of drinking, Roger is not getting the good feelings alcohol used to give him. He's having blackouts and memory problems. Anxiety and depression aren't relieved by alcohol any more but he can't quit drinking. His cravings are enormous if he stops drinking, even for only an hour or so. The last time he tried to quit drinking, he had a seizure.

Alcohol worked to lift Roger's spirits for awhile but now the depression is a constant companion, once again. Roger's depression and addiction to alcohol was the result of primary RDS.

NOTE: All five of these alcohol dependent people drink coffee and caffeinated beverages, eat large amounts of refined sugars and/or smoke tobacco. (Glen chews tobacco.) They are all hypoglycemic.

# DEPRESSION UNCOVERED

*No amount of talk therapy
will bring brain chemicals into balance.*

Depression comes in many forms. It can be normal depression which develops in response to stressful circumstances or it can be chronic depression that is ongoing, regardless of circumstances. It can be worried and anxious or flat, bored and apathetic. It can result from feeling overwhelmed and pressured or from being overly sensitive. Depression has many faces and many different causes and is a common side effect of addictions. It is often an underlying cause leading to self-medicating with alcohol.

If depression is an issue for you or someone you care about, I recommend reading my book *"Why Do I Feel This Way?" Natural Relief from Moods and Depression* before agreeing to take any prescription medications. (Available at www.BrainworksRecovery.com.)

Biochemical replacement therapy is not new. Over sixty years of research and experience have gone into the remarkable recoveries we are seeing today using all-natural resources without the use of prescription medications. Experts in this field are listed in Appendix C and I encourage you to delve into the mass of information and research on the internet, as well.

## SEVEN KINDS OF ALCOHOLIC DEPRESSION

Joan Mathews-Larson, PhD, founder and director of *Health Recovery Center* in Minneapolis, MN, has identified seven sources of biochemical depression affecting alcoholics and I refer to them here with a few comments about each.

## 1. NEUROTRANSMITTER DEPLETION  (See Chapter 19.)

This depletion stems from the inability to metabolize amino acids in the diet. (Alcohol *destroys* amino acids.) Due to the inherited genetic coding, Reward Deficiency Syndrome, the normal amount of amino acids is already decreased and alcohol consumption further reduces the supply.

Amino replacement therapy (more than 100 amino acids are in the body) is essential for recovery, along with abstinence from alcohol. Amino acid replacement is safe in most cases because the amino acids that are not needed by the body are rapidly excreted through the urine. (See precautions in Chapter 20.)

## SYMPTOMS OF AMINO ACID DEPLETION  (See Chapter 21.)

- anxiety
- high stress, tension
- depression
- short-term memory loss
- fatigue
- insomnia
- tremors, shakes
- irritability, sudden anger, violent outbursts,
- poor concentration,
- high distractibility

## 2. INBORN DEFICIENCY IN OMEGA-6 ESSENTIAL FATTY ACID (EFA)

Due to a genetic inability to metabolize Omega-6 fatty acid, there is a failure to manufacture enough prostaglandin E1 which is derived from essential fatty acids. Chronic childhood depression is the result. Alcohol stimulates temporary production of PGE1 and lifts the depression but when drinking is stopped, PGE1 production stops and depression returns. Using a biochemical approach, recovery from depression often occurs as early as three weeks into treatment. RDS, again. Essential fatty acids, along with the B vitamins, are necessary for the neurotransmitters to function properly. Today, this condition is rare in the U.S. Most people have too much Omega-6 and too little Omega-3.

## 3. VITAMIN/MINERAL DEFICIENCY  (See Chapter 22.)

Alcohol flushes many nutrients from the body and reduces the body's ability to metabolize foods properly, even if one is eating a healthy diet! As an example, let's consider the B vitamins. (Vitamin B's include a collection of vitamins that may not be related to each other and have different names.) They control nerve circuitry and are essential for the neurotransmitters to be used and distributed properly. These vitamins are destroyed by alcohol and by refined sugars, nicotine and caffeine, as well. (These substances are commonly consumed by alcoholics almost to the exclusion of anything else.) It's obvious why alcoholics are malnourished and why a healthy nutritional program is necessary for recovery.

## DEFICIENCY RESULT

| | |
|---|---|
| B1  Thiamine | Memory loss, central-nervous system damage, numbness and tingling in the arms and legs, mental confusion, nervousness, headache, poor concentration |
| B3  Niacin | Depression, fatigue, apprehension, headache, hyperactivity, insomnia |
| B5  Pantothenic Acid | Depression, irritability, tension, dizziness, moody, quarrelsome |

| B6   Pyridoxine | Anxiety, nervousness, depression, convulsions, extreme nervous exhaustion |
| --- | --- |
| Folic Acid | Agitation, moodiness, headaches, depression, fatigue, decreased sex drive |
| B12 | Lack of concentration, impulsive, angry, decreased memory, depression |
| Choline | Poor memory, gastric ulcers, high blood pressure, cardiac symptoms,  kidney/liver impairment |
| Inositol | Irritability, mood swings, panic attacks, obsessive-compulsive behavior arteriosclerosis, constipation, hair loss, high blood cholesterol, skin eruptions |

## 4. HYPOTHYROIDISM  (See Chapter 9.)

Hypothyroidism is due to an underactive thyroid that affects metabolism and creates multiple symptoms. Individuals should have a thyroid function test performed by their health care provider. (Thyroid medication should not be discontinued without a health care provider's consent.)

## SYMPTOMS OF HYPOTHYROIDISM

(Low Thyroid Function)
- depression
- mental sluggishness
- confusion
- poor memory
- fatigue
- low sex drive
- brittle hair
- dry skin
- puffiness around the eyes
- cold hands and feet
- sleeping more than eight hours a night
- susceptibility to colds and infections

## 5. FOOD AND CHEMICAL ALLERGIES  (See Chapter 26.)

Wheat and dairy are the most common food allergies. Alcoholics who are allergic to wheat drink in order to avoid their allergy symptoms, which are far too numerous to mention here. Allergy symptoms to chemicals and/or airborne substances such as molds, pollens, and fumes are often relieved by drinking alcohol, which, of course, is not the best solution. Relapse can be due to failure to diagnose and treat allergies.

In 2010, 3.93 billion pounds of toxic chemicals were released into the environment, up 16% from the year before. OSHA reports there are more than 100,000 Material Safety Data Sheets (MSDS) for toxic chemical substances. [1] (*Health Recovery Center* study showed that 56 percent of their clients were sensitive to chemicals in the environment.)[2]

From cosmetics to cleaning products, pesticides to environmental and airborne toxins, our bodies are assaulted 24 hours a day. For people who are sensitive to these chemicals, alcohol can sometimes provide temporary relief which can lead to an *acquired* Reward Deficiency Syndrome.

## 6. CANDIDA-RELATED COMPLEX  (See Chapter 26.)

Candida is a yeast overgrowth in the intestine that causes multiple symptoms including an intense craving for alcohol and refined sugars. Failure to address this complication will almost invariably lead to an early relapse.

(Pilot studies conducted at *Health Recovery Center* with 213 patients showed that 55 percent of the women and 35 percent of the men had histories indicating probable Candida overgrowth.)[3]

## 7. HYPOGLYCEMIA  (See Chapter 8.)

Hypoglycemia (low blood sugar due to an excess of insulin) is responsible for cravings and multiple symptoms which, if not addressed, lead to relapse. Removing refined sugars and caffeine, plus following a low-carbohydrate nutritional plan, can quickly relieve these symptoms.

## SYMPTOMS OF HYPOGLYCEMIA

These symptoms are identical to Chronic Abstinence Symptoms (Dry Drunk Syndrome)!!!

- nervousness
- irritability
- exhaustion
- rapid pulse
- depression
- drowsiness
- insomnia

- mental confusion
- constant worrying
- internal trembling
- forgetfulness
- headaches
- unprovoked anxieties

## SUMMARY

Multiple studies indicate that 88% to 95% of alcohol dependent people are hypoglycemic. Dr. Kenneth Williams, M.D., was an internist at the University of Pittsburgh, School of Medicine and a member of the National Board of Trustees of Alcoholics Anonymous. Williams has found that a vast majority of his sober alcohol dependent patients are hypoglycemic.[4] Abram Hoffer, MD and orthomolecular pioneer tested over 300 alcoholics. *All* were hypoglycemic.

After years of research, John Tintera, M.D. concluded that even recovered alcoholics who have been sober for many years continue to suffer from the effects of hypoglycemia. He strongly believes that the treatment of alcoholism "centers essentially about control [of hypoglycemia]".[5]

Tintera and other researchers who have documented the close connection between alcoholism and hypoglycemia consider *psychoanalytic treatment "utterly unsuccessful {in rehabilitating alcoholics} since the deep-rooted emotional factor is, in reality, physiologically based."*

As an RN in a hospital-based medical detoxification unit, as well as in other alcohol treatment facilities, I observed patients consuming enormous amounts of sugar filled colas, ice cream, French fried potatoes, chips, white breads and candy. The patients frequently ordered double portions of desserts. And, yes, they had all the symptoms of hypoglycemia including depression, mood swings, headaches, cravings, anxiety, fear and irritabilty.[6]

Jurriaan Plesman, Clinical Nutritionist, stated in an interview, "If you want to treat a dysfunctional family, you first have to treat them metabolically before you can help them with anything else. You can't reform a dysfunctional family if they all suffer from hypoglycemia."[7]

Except for hypothyroidism, which requires medication, all of these sources of alcoholic depression are relieved with proper nutrition and biochemical restoration; no medications required.

# PART TWO

## *SELF-TESTING*

# FINDING THE UNDERLYING CAUSE

The following tests will help to determine if there are any underlying contributing factors to your addiction in addition to a reward deficiency.[1] Attempting to relieve alcoholism without addressing these factors makes recovery difficult and usually ends up in relapse. Perhaps the most important test is the Hypothyroid test. If the thyroid is not operating properly, metabolism of supplements and foods will be poor and recovery will be doubtful. Having said that, all the tests are important and the results need to be addressed.

## TESTING

1. Follow the directions given with each test.
2. Answer the questions according to how you feel NOW, not how you felt in the past.
3. If you are questioning whether a symptom is true for you, it probably isn't important. If you have a symptom, you know it. It's experienced frequently or most of the time. We all have some symptoms, some of the time but they are not a problem.
4. Write down your scores at the end of each test, and also on the Total Accumulated Score page in Chapter 16.

Suggestions for follow-up are given at the end of each test. In some cases, your scores may indicate a need for further testing. If so, you will be advised to see a health care provider, however, many of these conditions can be effectively reversed with the combination of an appropriate nutritional diet and the right micronutrients and food supplements.

In case you may be inclined to skip these tests and just dive into repair, please think again. If any of these underlying issues are present and not addressed, recovery will be uncertain, at best.

# ALCOHOL SCREENING

Developed in 1971, the MICHIGAN ALCOHOL SCREENING TEST, (MAST), is one of the oldest and most accurate alcohol screening tests available. It identifies dependent drinkers with up to 98% accuracy.

The MAST test is a simple, self-scoring test that helps assess if you have a drinking problem. Answer "yes" or "no" to the following:

1. ___ Yes ___ No    Do you feel you are a normal drinker ("normal" is defined as drinking as much as, or less than, most other people)?

2. ___ Yes ___ No    Have you ever awakened the morning after drinking the night before and found that you could not remember a part of the evening?

3. ___ Yes ___ No    Does any near relative or close friend ever worry or complain about your drinking?

4. ___ Yes ___ No    Can you stop drinking without difficulty after one or two drinks?

5. ___ Yes ___ No    Do you ever feel guilty about your drinking?

6. ___ Yes ___ No    Have you ever attended a meeting of Alcoholics Anonymous (AA)?

7. ___ Yes ___ No    Have you ever gotten into physical fights when drinking?

8. ___ Yes ___ No    Has drinking ever created problems between you and a near relative or close friend?

9. ___ Yes ___ No    Has any family member or close friend gone to anyone for help about your drinking?

## MICHIGAN ALCOHOL SCREENING TEST continued

10. ___ Yes ___ No      Have you ever lost friends because of your drinking?

11. ___ Yes ___ No      Have you ever gotten into trouble at work because of drinking?

12. ___ Yes ___ No      Have you ever lost a job because of drinking?

13. ___ Yes ___ No      Have you ever neglected your obligations, family, or work for two or more days in a row because you were drinking?

14. ___ Yes ___ No      Do you drink before noon fairly often?

15. ___ Yes ___ No      Have you ever been told you have liver trouble, such as cirrhosis?

16. ___ Yes ___ No      After heavy drinking, have you ever had delirium tremens (DTs), severe shaking, visual or auditory (hearing) hallucinations?

17. ___ Yes ___ No      Have you ever gone to anyone for help about your drinking?

18. ___ Yes ___ No      Have you ever been hospitalized because of drinking?

19. ___ Yes ___ No      Has your drinking ever resulted in your being hospitalized in a mental health facility?

20. ___ Yes ___ No      Have you ever gone to any doctor, social worker, clergy person, or mental health clinic for help with any emotional problem in which drinking was part of the problem?

21. ___ Yes ___ No      Have you been arrested more than once for driving under the influence of alcohol?

22. ___ Yes ___ No      Have you ever been arrested, or detained by an official for a few hours, because of other behavior while drinking?

SCORE one point each if you answered "no" to questions 1 and 4. _____

SCORE one point each if you answered "yes" to questions 2, 3, and 5 through 22. _____

TOTAL SCORE _____

A **total score of six or more** indicates hazardous drinking or alcohol dependence and further evaluation by a healthcare professional is recommended. This includes reversing the condition immediately by getting the appropriate help.

# CARBOHYDRATE ADDICTION

It's difficult to avoid the bad (simple) carbohydrates. Sugar, in many forms, is found in all processed foods, very often as a first or second ingredient. Excess sugar is a poison, four times more addictive than cocaine.

American's love affair with the "whites" (flour, rice, pasta, potatoes, etc.) continues to grow. And now, the food industry is regularly including chemicals in foods that stimulate the appetite. 35.7% of Americans are obese (20% over normal weight) and 68% are overweight (20 or more pounds above normal weight).

11.3% of people over age 20 and 26.9% of people over age 65 have diabetes and the number is climbing as Americans make sugar and simple carbohydrates their number-one foods of choice.

While most of us consume some level of sugars, and other simple carbohydrates, not everyone is addicted to it, though most are. An addiction creates symptoms of dis-ease in all its forms. Take this test to find out if you are addicted to simple carbohydrates.

_____ 1. When eating sweets, starches, or snack foods, do you find it hard to stop?

_____ 2. At a restaurant, do you eat several rolls or bread before the meal is served?

_____ 3. While eating carbohydrates, do you ever feel out of control?

_____ 4. Does your diet consist mainly of breads, pastas, starchy vegetables, fast foods, and/or sweets?

_____ 5. Do you ever hide food or eat food secretly?

_____ 6. Do you binge on snack foods, candy, or fast foods?

_____ 7. Does eating a sweet snack lift your spirits?

_____ 8. Do you feel hungry and unsatisfied after a meal no matter how much you eat?

# CARBOHYDRATE ADDICTION TEST continued

_____ 9.  Do you feel sleepy or groggy after a high-carbohydrate meal (i.e., breads, potatoes, pastas, dessert)?

_____ 10.  Which would you prefer?

| | | |
|---|---|---|
| ____ breaded fish | or | ____ baked fish |
| ____ potato | or | ____ broccoli |
| ____ sandwich | or | ____ salad |
| ____ chips | or | ____ raw nuts |
| ____ cookie | or | ____ strawberries |
| ____ cracker | or | ____ raw vegetables |
| ____ spaghetti | or | ____ steak |

(For question 10, consider your response a "yes" if you checked more items in the left-hand column than in the right-hand column.)

Total the number of "yes" responses to these ten questions. Then determine which of the following categories you fit into:

TOTAL SCORE: _____

1-2   Doubtful Addiction

3-4   Mild Addiction

5-6   Moderate Addiction

7-10 Severe Addiction

If your score is over 5, you will benefit by restricting your carbohydrates to fifty to seventy-five grams daily. Follow the LOW CARBOHYDRATE FOOD PLAN in Chapter 25 for three to four weeks, then shift to the OPTIMAL HEALTH FOOD PLAN.

In almost all cases, your weight will shift toward normal in a healthy and gradual manner. Many symptoms of dis-ease will simply disappear.

Adapted from *Seven Weeks to Sobriety – Joan Mathews Larson, Ph.D.*

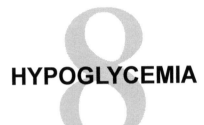

# HYPOGLYCEMIA

Hypoglycemia, or low blood sugar, is an abnormally diminished amount of glucose in the blood. The term literally means "low sugar blood". It can produce a variety of symptoms and effects but the principal problems arise from an inadequate supply of glucose to the brain, resulting in impairment of function.

Effects can range from mild mental and emotional experiences of depression, discontent and indifference to the world around one to more serious issues such as seizures, unconsciousness, and (rarely) permanent brain damage or death.

## SYMPTOMS OF HYPOGLYCEMIA

Place a check mark in front of any or all the symptoms you frequently experience.

| | |
|---|---|
| _____ Nervousness | _____ Internal trembling |
| _____ Anxiety | _____ Forgetfulness |
| _____ Irritability | _____ Headaches |
| _____ Indecisiveness | _____ Hunger |
| _____ Exhaustion | _____ Sighing or yawning |
| _____ Weakness | _____ Craving for sweetness or alcohol |
| _____ Rapid pulse | _____ Faintness |
| _____ Sweating | _____ Dizziness |

_____ Heart palpitations                _____ Uncoordinated

_____ Depression                        _____ Double vision

_____ Drowsiness                        _____ Blurred vision

_____ Leg cramps                        _____ Tremor

_____ Unprovoked anxieties              _____ Seizures

_____ Insomnia                          _____ Suicidal thoughts

_____ Numbness                          _____ Loss of consciousness

_____ Crying spells                     _____ Unprovoked anxieties

_____ Mental confusion                  _____ Muscle twitching or jerking

_____ Abnormal behavior                 _____ Itching and crawling skin sensations

_____ Constant worrying                 _____ Tingling sensation around the mouth

## HYPOGLYCEMIA TOTAL SCORE _____

If you tested positive for a Carbohydrate Addiction (Chapter 4), you are most likely also hypoglycemic. 95% to 100% of alcoholics are hypoglycemic, but then, so are most Americans.

Hypoglycemia creates strong cravings for sugar which is in all processed food, junk food, and sodas. Food cravings, obesity and diabetes are directly related to hypoglycemia. Alcohol rapidly converts to sugar. Tobacco is cured in sugar. With the aid of a good supplement and nutritional program, this condition can be reversed.

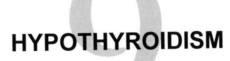

# HYPOTHYROIDISM

The thyroid gland makes two primary hormones, T3 and T4. The T stands for the amino acid Tyrosine and the 3 and 4 stand for the number of iodine molecules in each hormone. These two hormones ignite every cell of your body and brain by activating its genetic coding. Without proper thyroid function, the neurotransmitters can't alter your moods effectively.

Everyone should have a thyroid function test on a regular basis. Certainly, if your thyroid function is less than normal and left untreated, proper nutrition and supplementation, while helpful, will not provide you the rewards you hope for.

There are three kinds of thyroid diseases. Graves Disease and hyPERthyroidism. However, the most common thyroid malfunction is hyPOthyroidism. If your moods, depression, or other symptoms are caused by hypothyroidism, you'll want to know about it and correct the condition.

## RISK FACTORS FOR HYPOTHYROIDISM INCLUDE (BUT ARE NOT LIMITED TO):

- Family history of thyroid disease
- History of another autoimmune disease
- Had a baby in the past nine months
- History of miscarriage

## SYMPTOMS OF HYPOTHYROIDISM

Check all symptoms you frequently experience.

_____ Gaining weight inappropriately

_____ Unable to lose weight with diet/exercise

# HYPOTHYROIDISM continued

_____ Constipated, sometimes severely

_____ Hypothermia/low body temperature (Feel cold when others feel hot, need extra sweaters, etc.)

_____ Fatigued, exhausted

_____ Run down, sluggish, lethargic

_____ Hair is coarse and dry, breaking, brittle, falling out

_____ Skin is coarse, dry, scaly, and thick

_____ Hoarse or gravely voice

_____ Puffiness and swelling around the eyes and face

_____ Pains, aches in joints, hands and feet

_____ Carpal-tunnel syndrome

_____ Irregular menstrual cycles (longer, or heavier, or more frequent)

_____ Trouble conceiving a baby

_____ Depressed

_____ Restless

_____ Moods change easily

_____ Feelings of worthlessness

_____ Difficulty concentrating

_____ Feelings of sadness

_____ Losing interest in normal daily activities

_____ More forgetful lately

_____ Hair is falling out

_____ Can't seem to remember things

# HYPOTHYROIDISM continued

_____ No sex drive

_____ Getting more frequent infections, that last longer

_____ Snoring more lately

_____ Have or may have sleep apnea

_____ Shortness of breath and tightness in the chest

_____ Feel the need to yawn to get oxygen

_____ Eyes feel gritty and dry

_____ Eyes feel sensitive to light

_____ Eyes get jumpy/tics in eyes creating dizziness/vertigo and headaches

_____ Strange feelings in neck or throat

_____ Tinnitus (ringing in ears)

_____ Recurrent sinus infections

_____ Vertigo

_____ Lightheadedness

_____ Menstrual cramps

## TOTAL NUMBER OF CHECKS _____

If you have several of these symptoms, inform your healthcare provider, and get a lab test, and medication if appropriate. Natural thyroid supplementation does not usually provide consistent dependable quality. We recommend prescription medication which is inexpensive and works very well.

LABORATORY TESTING: I recommend getting TSH, Free T3 and Free T4 testing. Your physician may not want to do the Free T3 and Free T4 tests. They are far more accurate than the T3 and T4. If your physician refuses, see testing resources in Appendix B.

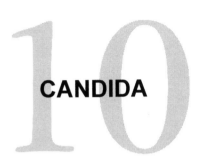

# CANDIDA

Thirty million plus people suffer from an *overgrowth* of *candida* and that's only the number in North America. Roughly half the world's population will suffer from a candida-related condition in their lifetime.

Candida is a type of yeast fungus normally found among the balance of "good" and "bad" bacteria in a healthy person's digestive system. It lives in 80% of the human population without causing harmful effects. The intestine's friendly flora, lactobacilli acidophilus, bifidophilus, and others usually keep Candida in check but when there is an overgrowth of the candida yeast many symptoms can develop. Because the yeast lives on sugar, it will cause irresistible cravings making it difficult to stop addictions to alcohol, drugs, and sweet foods.

The person with candida overgrowth may be walking through life quite ill with the following experiences:

- ✓ All laboratory tests come back "normal".
- ✓ You're being treated for various ailments whose symptoms return when the medication is finished, possibly with additional side effects and no resolution.
- ✓ You've been told your symptoms are "psychological".
- ✓ You are misdiagnosed and incorrectly treated, worsening your health challenges.

An overgrowth of Candida yeast blocks proper digestion and elimination. It robs the body of vitamins, minerals and other nutrients from both food and supplements. It spreads from the gut to genitals, oral cavities and mucous membranes, pouring toxins into the blood and eventually affecting various organs in the body. In short, *candida eats what you eat, and when there is no nutrition left, it nourishes itself on your muscles and bones.* Where it can't eat, it causes deterioration.

Therefore, candida is tied into many of our chronic ailments and can create a miserable situation for its host if not caught and treated. Enough said.

# CANDIDA continued

**Section A: History**

_____1. Have you taken tetracycline's or other antibiotics for acne for 1 month (or longer)? Give yourself 35 points

_____2. Have you at any time in your life taken broad-spectrum antibiotics or other antibacterial medications for respiratory, urinary or other infections for two months or longer, or in shorter courses four or more times in one year? 35 points

_____3. Have you taken a broad-spectrum antibiotic drug - even in a single dose? 6 points

_____4. Have you at any time in your life, been bothered by persistent prostatitis, vaginitis, or other problems affecting your reproductive organs? 25 points

_____5. Are you bothered by memory or concentration problems? Do you sometimes feel spaced out? 20 points

_____6. Do you feel "sick all over" yet, in spite of visits to many different physicians, the causes have not been found? 20 points

_____7. Have you been pregnant...2 or more times?  5 points   ...one time?  3 points

_____8. Have you taken birth control pills... for more than two years? 15 points ... for six months to two years? 8 points

_____9. Have you taken steroids orally, by injection or inhalation... for more than two weeks? 15 points ....for two weeks or less? 6 points

_____10. Does exposure to perfumes, insecticides, and other chemicals provoke moderate to severe symptoms? 20 points .... mild symptoms? 5 points

_____11. Does tobacco smoke really bother you? 10 points

_____12. Are your symptoms worse on damp, muggy days, or in moldy places? 20 points

_____13. Have you had athlete's foot, ring worm, jock itch, or other chronic fungal infections of the skin or nails? Have such infections been... severe or persistent? 20 points ... mild to moderate? 10 points

_____14. Do you crave sugar? 10 points

Total Score, Section A _____

# CANDIDA continued

**Section B: Major Symptoms**
Does not apply=0 points
Mild or occasional=3 points
Moderate or frequent=6 points
Severe or disabling=9 points

_____ 1. Fatigue or lethargy

_____ 2. Feeling drained

_____ 3. Depression or manic depression

_____ 4. Numbness, burning or tingling

_____ 5. Headache

_____ 6. Muscle aches

_____ 7. Muscle weakness or paralysis

_____ 8. Pain and/or swelling in joints

_____ 9. Abdominal pain

_____10. Constipation and/or diarrhea

_____11. Bloating, belching or intestinal gas

_____12. Vaginal burning, itching or discharge

_____13. Prostatitis

_____14. Impotence

_____15. Loss of sexual desire or feeling

_____16. Endometriosis or infertility

_____17. Cramps and/or other menstrual irregularities

_____18. Premenstrual tension

# CANDIDA continued

_____19. Attacks of anxiety or crying

_____20. Cold hands or feet, low body temperature

_____21. Hypothyroidism

_____22. Shaking or irritable when hungry

_____23. Cystitis or interstitial cystitis (bladder inflammation)

Total Score, Section B _____

**Section C, Other Symptoms**
Does not apply=0 points
Mild or occasional=1 point
Moderate or frequent=2 points
Severe or disabling=3 points

_____ 1. Drowsiness, including inappropriate drowsiness

_____ 2. Irritability

_____ 3. Uncoordinated

_____ 4. Frequent mood swings

_____ 5. Insomnia

_____ 6. Dizziness/loss of balance

_____ 7. Pressure above ears... feeling of head swelling

_____ 8. Sinus problems... tenderness of cheekbones or forehead

_____ 9. Tendency to bruise easily

_____10. Eczema, itching eyes

_____11. Psoriasis

_____12. Chronic hives (urticaria)

_____13. Indigestion or heartburn

# CANDIDA continued

_____14. Sensitivity to milk, wheat, corn or other common foods

_____15. Mucus in stools

_____16. Spots in front of eyes or erratic vision _____17. Burning or tearing eyes

_____18. Recurrent infections or fluid in ears

_____19. Ear pain or deafness

Total Score, Section C _____

Score, Section A _____

Score, Section B _____

Score, Section C _____

**Grand Total Score** _____

## RESULTS
If your score is MORE THAN 180 in women and MORE THAN 140 in men, systemic yeast is **almost certainly** present.

If your score is MORE THAN 120 in women and MORE THAN 90 in men, systemic yeast is **probably** present.

If your score is MORE THAN 60 in women and MORE THAN 40 in men, systemic yeast is **possibly** present.

With scores LESS THAN 60 in women and LESS THAN 40 in men, systemic yeast is **less likely** to cause health problems.

This questionnaire is taken from *The Yeast Connection Handbook*, by William G. Crook, MD. 1999

Candida can sometimes be cured with non-prescription supplements, however you may need to use a prescription such as Diflucan, especially if you have a very bad case. There are homeopathic products that can eliminate candida, as well. It's important to eliminate junk foods, sugars, pastas, and white flour products from the diet, and to take food supplements, including a B vitamin complex. (See Chapter 26 for more information.)

# 11
# FOOD ALLERGIES

Whole grain wheat bread is good for us, right? Maybe. Maybe we eat it as toast for breakfast, in a sandwich for lunch, and as bread or rolls with dinner. We don't associate our fatigue or insomnia with healthy bread, but these and other symptoms we're experiencing may be the result of an allergy to wheat or gluten. In addition, some alcohol addicted people are actually allergic to the wheat, barley, rye, and rice that are used to make their alcoholic drinks. To find out if you are allergic to foods, you can use a simple test that can be done at home.

Allergies are far more common than most people think and are the cause of so many symptoms. The good news is that once the allergy is detected, by eliminating the offending food from one's diet, the symptoms are relieved. No more suffering and no more prescription medications to cover up the symptoms. (One can occasionally eat the offending food later.) The most common allergens are 1) wheat and its cousins - rye, barley, and oats, and 2) cow's milk products including milk, cheese or anything else made from the modern cow. Runners-up are soy and the nightshade family (tomatoes, peppers, white potatoes, eggplant, and tobacco). Runners-up, especially for children, are chocolate, corn, peanuts, eggs, oranges, and foods high in salicylates like apples.[1]

Do you crave it? Eat it daily? Don't want to give it up? These are clues. Listed below are some allergy related disorders.

- Attention deficit
- Bronchial asthma
- Bronchitis
- Chronic diarrhea
- Chronic fatigue syndrome
- Depression
- Headaches (migraine and non-migraine)
- Hyperactivity
- Insomnia
- Learning disorders
- Sleep disorders
- Tension-fatigue syndrome

# FOOD ALLERGIES continued

ALLERGY SYMPTOMS    Check all symptoms that apply to you.

_____ Irritability

_____ Angry outbursts

_____ Glum lethargy

_____ Teary eyes

_____ Hyperactivity

_____ Stress

_____ Depression

_____ Asthma

_____ Sore throat

_____ Earaches

_____ Stuffy nose

_____ Postnasal drip

_____ Constipation

_____ Diarrhea

_____ Stomachache

_____ Bloat

_____ Gas

_____ Reflux

_____ Heartburn

_____ Low energy

_____ Sleepiness (especially right after meals)

# FOOD ALLERGIES continued

_____ Joint pain

_____ Achiness

_____ Poor concentration

_____ Addictive cravings for the allergy food or for sweets

_____ **TOTAL SYMPTOM SCORE**  A high score may indicate allergies.

## INSTRUCTIONS

1.  Complete the first four questions.
2.  In Question Five, Food Questionnaire, **circle any foods** you listed in Question Three.
3.  Women only: In Question Five **circle any foods** you listed in Question Four.
4.  In Question Five, circle any heading above a section that contains foods eaten six or seven days per week.

## SCREENING TEST FOR FOOD ALLERGIES

1.  List a typical day's meals and snacks:

    | BREAKFAST | LUNCH | DINNER | SNACKS |
    |---|---|---|---|
    | | | | |
    | | | | |
    | | | | |
    | | | | |
    | | | | |

2.  List your three most favorite foods that you eat regularly.

    _____

3.  Do you crave or binge on any foods?  If so, which ones?

    _____

4.  (For women)  Do you crave or binge on foods premenstrually?  If so, which ones?

    _____

5.  Food Questionnaire
    How many days in one week do you eat the following foods:  (Write the number of days on the line following the food.)

## FOOD ALLERGIES continued

### WHEAT/YEAST

| | | | |
|---|---|---|---|
| Bread | ___ | Spaghetti | ___ |
| Rolls | ___ | Casseroles | ___ |
| Muffins | ___ | Pizza | ___ |
| Sandwiches | ___ | Breakfast cereal | ___ |
| Bagels | ___ | Crackers | ___ |
| Pasta | ___ | Cookies | ___ |
| Macaroni | ___ | Canned soup | ___ |
| Noodles | ___ | Pastries | ___ |

### CORN

| | | | |
|---|---|---|---|
| Popcorn | ___ | Cornflakes | ___ |
| Lunch meat | ___ | Corn (vegetable) | ___ |
| Tacos | ___ | Pancake syrup | ___ |

### OTHER GRAINS

| | | | |
|---|---|---|---|
| Rice | ___ | Other | ___ |
| Oatmeal | ___ | | |

### DAIRY

| | | | |
|---|---|---|---|
| Milk | ___ | Margarine | ___ |
| Cheese | ___ | Butter | ___ |
| Yogurt | ___ | Cream cheese | ___ |
| Ice cream | ___ | Cottage cheese | ___ |
| Coffee creamer | ___ | | |

### EGGS

| | | | |
|---|---|---|---|
| Scrambled, omelet, etc. | ___ | French toast | ___ |
| Mayonnaise | ___ | | |

### MISCELLANEOUS

| | | | |
|---|---|---|---|
| Vinegar | ___ | Prunes | ___ |
| Salad dressing | ___ | Ketchup | ___ |
| Mushrooms | ___ | Mustard | ___ |
| Soy sauce | ___ | Peanuts | ___ |
| Raisons | ___ | Other nuts | ___ |
| Dates | ___ | | |

# FOOD ALLERGIES continued

## DESSERT

| | | | |
|---|---|---|---|
| Jell-0 | ____ | Sweet 'N Low | ____ |
| Jelly/jam | ____ | Equal | ____ |
| | | NutraSweet | ____ |

## BEEF

| | | | |
|---|---|---|---|
| Beef roast | ____ | Steak | ____ |
| Hamburger | ____ | | |

## PORK

| | | | |
|---|---|---|---|
| Ham | ____ | Sausage | ____ |
| Bacon | ____ | Pork chops | ____ |

## OTHER PROTEIN

| | | | |
|---|---|---|---|
| Chicken | ____ | _____ | ____ |
| Turkey | ____ | _____ | ____ |
| Fish | ____ | Soy/tofu | ____ |
| _____ | ____ | Hot dogs | ____ |

## BEVERAGES

| | | | |
|---|---|---|---|
| Diet soda | ____ | Coffee | ____ |
| Alcoholic beverages | ____ | Tea | ____ |
| Soda _____ | ____ | Fruit juice | ____ |

## SNACKS

| | | | |
|---|---|---|---|
| Potato chips | ____ | Chocolate | ____ |

## FRUIT

| | | | |
|---|---|---|---|
| Apples | ____ | Grapes | ____ |
| Bananas | ____ | Pineapple | ____ |
| Oranges | ____ | Other: | |
| Pears | ____ | _____ | ____ |
| Melon | ____ | _____ | ____ |
| Grapefruit | ____ | | |

# FOOD ALLERGIES continued

## VEGETABLES

| | | | |
|---|---|---|---|
| Tomato | ____ | Broccoli | ____ |
| Green pepper | ____ | Cabbage/coleslaw | ____ |
| Peas | ____ | Cauliflower | ____ |
| Green beans | ____ | Other: | |
| Other beans: | | | |
| | | _____ | ____ |
| _____ | ____ | Lettuce salads | ____ |
| Carrots | ____ | Potatoes/French fries | ____ |
| Celery | ____ | | |

## SPICES

| | | | |
|---|---|---|---|
| Onion | ____ | Ginger | ____ |
| Garlic | ____ | Parsley | ____ |
| Pepper | ____ | Oregano | ____ |
| Dry mustard | ____ | Cinnamon | ____ |
| Basil | ____ | Mint | ____ |
| Paprika | ____ | Other:____ | ____ |
| Rosemary | ____ | _____ | ____ |

## INSTRUCTIONS repeated:

1.  Complete the first four questions.
2.  In Question Five, Food Questionnaire, circle any foods you listed in Question Three.
3.  Women only: In Question Five circle any foods you listed in Question Four.
4.  In Question Five, circle any heading above a section that contains foods eaten six or seven days per week.

## LIST THE FOODS YOU HAVE CIRCLED IN QUESTION FIVE

_____

_____

_____

_____

The foods you have circled and listed above are the ones most likely to trigger addictive cravings and delayed allergic reactions. Allergic reactions occur within minutes to forty eight hours after eating the offending food. That's why we wait 72 hours before testing a second food.

The most effective test for food allergies is the elimination diet. This test is fully explained in Chapter 26.

*This self-screening test was designed by George Kroker, M.D.*

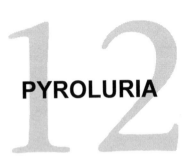

# PYROLURIA

Pyroluria is the result of a genetically-caused over-production of a group of chemicals called kyrptopyrroles. These pyrroles bind with B6 and zinc and dump them into the urine which is then excreted from the body creating emotional disaster. A high incidence of Pyrrole Disorder is found in individuals on the autism spectrum, individuals with anxiety disorder, depression, obsessive-compulsive disorder, schizophrenia, bipolar disorder, Aspergers, AD(H)D, and alcoholism (44%). However, pyroluria is quickly and easily corrected when diagnosed.

## MAJOR INDICATIONS

Check "yes" or "no" for each of the questions below.

YES  NO

___ ___     Do you sunburn easily?  Do you have fair or pale skin?

___ ___     Do you tend to avoid stressful situations?

___ ___     Do you have poor dream recall or only exciting dreams (nightmares)?

___ ___     Is it hard to recall what you've just read?

___ ___     Are your eyes sensitive to bright lights?

___ ___     Do you get frequent colds or infections?

___ ___     Are there white spots/flecks on your fingernails?

___ ___     Are you prone to acne, eczema, or psoriasis?

## PYROLURIA continued

YES   NO

—— ——    Do you have stretch marks on your skin?

—— ——    Do you prefer not to eat breakfast or even experience light nausea in the morning?

—— ——    Are there severe mood problems, mental illness, or alcoholism in your family?

SCORE  YES ANSWERS _____

## INDICATIONS THAT ARE OCCASIONALLY PRESENT

YES   NO

—— ——    Do you have a reduced amount of head hair or do you have prematurely gray hair?

—— ——    Are you becoming more of a loner as you age?

—— ——    Have you been anxious, fearful, or felt a lot of inner tension since childhood?

—— ——    If you are over age 16, do you have bouts of depression and/or nervous exhaustion?

—— ——    Do you have headaches?

—— ——    Did you reach puberty earlier or later than normal?

—— ——    Do you sneeze in sunlight?

—— ——    Do loud noises bother you?

—— ——    Do you prefer the company of one or two close friends rather than a gathering of friends?

—— ——    Have you noticed a sweet smell (fruity odor) to your breath or sweat when ill or stressed? (Rare symptom)

—— ——    Do you have a poor appetite or a poor sense of taste?  Do you enjoy spicy food?

—— ——    Do you have any upper abdominal or spleen pain?  As a child, did you get a "stitch" in your side when you ran?  (1 in 10 have this symptom.)

—— ——    Do your knees crack or ache?

—— ——    Are you anemic?  (1 in 10 have this symptom)

—— ——    Are you easily upset (internally) by criticism?

# PYROLURIA continued

YES   NO

\_\_\_  \_\_\_    Do you have frequent mood swings?

\_\_\_  \_\_\_    Do you tend to carry any excess fat in your lower extremities rather than evenly distributed around your body (a pear-shaped figure)?

SCORE YES ANSWERS _____

If you have any of the disorders listed in the first part of this chapter and if you answered "yes" to FIVE or more of the MAJOR INDICATIONS and "yes" to *some* of the OCCASIONALLY PRESENT questions, you might want to consider getting a pyrrole urine test. For the location of recommended laboratory testing facilities go to Appendix B.

**This condition, if present, is 100% correctable with the proper micronutrients. Recovery can occur in a few weeks.**

© *2013 This questionnaire, originally developed by Carl Pfeiffer, PhD., has been updated by Suka Chapel-Horst, RN, PhD, in consultation with William J. Walsh, PhD.*

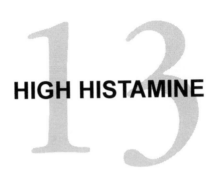

# HIGH HISTAMINE

Whole families can have high histamine levels. 75% of these include high achievers, great athletes, CEO's, MDs, or scientists. 20%, however, may have hyperactivity, depression, aggressiveness, obsessive/compulsive behavior, and a racing brain. They may grow obsessive about sex, cry easily, have abnormal fears, and contemplate suicide.

## DIRECTIONS

Check "yes" or "no" for each of the questions below.

| | YES | NO | |
|---|---|---|---|
| 1. | ____ | ____ | Do you tend to sneeze in bright sunlight? |
| 2. | ____ | ____ | Were you a shy and oversensitive teenager? |
| 3. | ____ | ____ | Can you make tears and saliva easily and never have a dry mouth? |
| 4. | ____ | ____ | Do you have a high sensitivity to pain? |
| 5. | ____ | ____ | Do you get headaches regularly? |
| 6. | ____ | ____ | Do you have seasonal allergies, such as hay fever?  (75%) |
| 7. | ____ | ____ | Do you need only five to seven hours of sleep each night? |
| 8. | ____ | ____ | Are you a perfectionist or an obsessive, Type-A personality who feels driven? |

SCORE YES ANSWERS _____

# HIGH HISTAMINE continued

If you have any of the disorders listed in the first part of this chapter and if you answered "yes" to FOUR or more of these questions, you might want to consider laboratory testing of your histamine level. For the location of recommended laboratory testing facilities go to Appendix B.

© *2013 This questionnaire, originally developed by Carl Pfeiffer, PhD., has been updated by Suka Chapel-Horst, RN, PhD, in consultation with William J. Walsh, PhD.*

# LOW HISTAMINE

Histamine is a major brain neurotransmitter that causes incredible chaos when it rises to abnormal highs or falls dangerously low. If people have too little histamine, they may experience panic, anxiety, sleep disorders, bipolar symptoms, suicidal thoughts, psychosis, or schizophrenia.

## MAJOR INDICATIONS

Check "yes" or "no" for each of the questions below.

| YES | NO | |
|-----|-----|---|
| ____ | ____ | Do you have slow sexual responsiveness or a low libido? (adults) |
| ____ | ____ | Do you have heavy growth of body hair? (adults) |
| ____ | ____ | Do you have a head full of grand plans but are easily frustrated? |
| ____ | ____ | Are you suspicious of people or do you feel paranoid? |
| ____ | ____ | Is your mouth usually dry? Do you have dry eyes? |
| ____ | ____ | Do you have a tendency to despair, or have bouts of crying? |

SCORE YES ANSWERS _____

## LOW HISTAMINE continued

## INDICATIONS THAT ARE OCCASIONALLY PRESENT

YES   NO

\_\_\_\_  \_\_\_\_    Do you get canker sores?

\_\_\_\_  \_\_\_\_    Do you have tension headaches or seldom have headaches?

\_\_\_\_  \_\_\_\_    Have you ever heard voices inside your head?

\_\_\_\_  \_\_\_\_    Are you able to stand pain well?

\_\_\_\_  \_\_\_\_    Do you get few or no colds?

\_\_\_\_  \_\_\_\_    Do you need at least eight hours of sleep, and are you a slow riser in the morning?

\_\_\_\_  \_\_\_\_    Do you experience frequent irritability?

SCORE YES ANSWERS _____

If you have any of the disorders listed in the first part of this chapter, and if you answered "yes" to FOUR or more of the MAJOR INDICATIONS and "yes" to **some** of the OCCASIONALLY PRESENT questions ask your Health Care Provider to order laboratory testing of both your histamine and copper levels. Excess copper destroys histamine in the brain. This can cause violent behavior and depression, as well as paranoia. For the location of recommended laboratory testing facilities go to Appendix B.

*© 2013 This questionnaire, originally developed by Carl Pfeiffer, PhD., has been updated by Suka Chapel-Horst, RN, PhD, in consultation with William J. Walsh, PhD.*

# 15
# ATTENTION DEFICIT
# (HYPERACTIVITY) DISORDER

I've included AD(H)D in this test manual because it's been estimated that between 40% to 70% of alcoholics have *undiagnosed* AD(H)D. If teenagers with AD(H)D find that alcohol reduces their symptoms, making life far easier and happier, then alcohol becomes a very "sweet" way to self-medicate.

When someone with AD(H)D stops drinking, the underlying AD(H)D symptoms return and, rather than decreasing over time, the symptoms become worse. This quickly leads to relapse in order to obtain welcome relief.

Unfortunately, the person is usually blamed for his failure to remain sober while the underlying cause goes undetected. (See Chapter 32 on PAWS.) This is unfair and unfortunate. While AD(H)D cannot be completed overturned, the symptoms can be greatly reduced and the person can learn how to live a successful and happy life. The guidelines in this program will assist in reducing symptoms of AD(H)D.

## Symptoms of Attention Deficit Disorder (ADD)

Check any symptoms that apply to you.

_____ Losing things

_____ Poor listener

_____ Easily distracted

_____ Poor organization

_____ Forgetful in daily activities

# ATTENTION DEFICIT (HYPERACTIVITY) DISORDER continued

\_\_\_\_\_ Lack of sustained attention

\_\_\_\_\_ Failure to follow through on tasks

\_\_\_\_\_ Careless mistakes/lack of attention to details

\_\_\_\_\_ Avoiding tasks requiring sustained mental effort

## SYMPTOMS OF ATTENTION DEFICIT HYPERACTIVITY DISORDER (ADHD)

ADHD is ADD with the addition of *hyperactivity.* The following are additional symptoms *plus* those of ADD. Check any symptoms that applied to you as a child and may still apply.

\_\_\_\_\_ Intrusive

\_\_\_\_\_ "On the go"

\_\_\_\_\_ Leaving your seat

\_\_\_\_\_ Can't wait your turn

\_\_\_\_\_ Excessive talking

\_\_\_\_\_ Fidgeting/squirming

\_\_\_\_\_ Blurting out answers

\_\_\_\_\_ Excessive running/climbing

\_\_\_\_\_ Difficulty with quiet activities

If these patterns are familiar, then getting psychological testing is warranted, *regardless of a person's age.* AD(H)D does not decrease as a person ages. People become more adjusted to it and learn methods of coping with it, but the disorder remains.

If the diagnosis is, indeed, AD(H)D, there is biochemical help. This disorder is not 100% correctable, however, the symptoms can be greatly reduced with the aid of biochemical treatment.

Be aware that pharmaceutical drugs used for AD(H)D symptoms, such as Ritalin, are highly addictive. (Ritalin is slower acting but more addictive than cocaine.) Most importantly, they do not relieve the underlying cause, which is an inherited, genetic Reward Deficiency. Research has shown that long-term use of drugs such as Ritalin usually makes the condition worse over time. Biochemical restoration can reduce the symptoms and improve concentration.

# TOTAL ACCUMULATED SCORES

16

You can place your scores from all the previous tests here for easy reference. As you move through your *recovery phase* you will find it helpful and encouraging to retake some of the tests and compare your later scores to the earlier ones.

TEST SCORES  Date _____          REDO TEST SCORES Date _____

_____ ALCOHOL SCREENING (Chapter 6)                _____

_____ CARBOHYDRATE ADDICTION (Chapter 7)           _____

_____ HYPOGLYCEMIA (Chapter 8)                     _____

_____ HYPOTHYROIDISM (Chapter 9)                   _____

_____ CANDIDA (Chapter 10)                         _____

_____ FOOD ALLERGIES (Chapter11)                   _____

_____ PYROLURIA (Chapter 12)                       _____

_____ HIGH HISTAMINE (Chapter 13)                  _____

_____ LOW HISTAMINE (Chapter 14)                   _____

For recommended laboratory testing go to Appendix B.

# PART THREE

## *PREPARATION*

# 17

# WHO CAN DO IT?

Are you wondering if you can benefit from this alcohol recovery program? Here are some typical questions.

## AM I AN ALCOHOLIC?

This is a question you may have been asking yourself, or perhaps you're reading this book to inform someone else or simply out of curiosity. Good for you.

Only about three percent of alcoholics attend Alcoholics Anonymous meetings for a variety of personal reasons. And, unless the disease of alcoholism has progressed to a point where family and friends become insistent about sending their loved one to a treatment program, or medical complications disrupt normal life, most individuals continue to deny that they have a drinking problem, or ignore it, or justify it, or drink in private, or attempt to keep it a secret hoping everything will soon get better, or there may be a combination of all of these.

Perhaps you are reluctant to admit to having a problem with alcohol. Remember, no shame, no blame, no guilt. It's simply a biochemical dysfunction that can be reversed. The MAST test in Chapter 6 is highly accurate. If you tested positive on this test, it's time to start your recovery program. If you have attempted to recover in the past and have relapsed, it was probably because the underlying cause, biochemical imbalances, was not addressed.

## WHO WILL BENEFIT FROM THIS PROGRAM?

You are appropriate for this program if you are a highly functioning individual and are:

- ready,
- willing,
- capable,
- motivated,
- determined, and
- you will do anything to get your life back.

Highly functioning means that you can follow a supplement schedule, purchase and prepare nutritious foods, (if a family member is not present who is helping you with this), schedule regular dry-heat, infra-red saunas and weekly massages for four to six weeks, exercise or walk four times a week, and are willing to create a personal support system to keep you on track with encouragement and assistance whenever you may need it. This may or may not include attendance at AA meetings. That is your choice, however a support system of some kind will be vital to your ongoing recovery.

## WHO SHOULD NOT DO THIS PROGRAM?

This program is NOT appropriate for individuals who have serious medical conditions, are on multiple medications, or have a diagnosed mental illness. In these cases, the amino acids should not be taken without the advice of a *qualified* healthcare provider. However, the nutritional portion of this program will be useful for most people. More specifically:

1. If you have heart disease, diabetes or a history of seizures, you should have your healthcare provider's approval before beginning this program. The nutritional portion of this program will be of great benefit to you and the amino acids may be taken with caution and monitoring.
2. If you are taking antidepressants, benzodiazepines, opiates, or stimulants, you will benefit from a biochemically oriented residential program that can assist you with tapering off these substances safely.
3. If you have high or low histamine levels, or pyroluria, laboratory testing and follow-up with a *qualified* healthcare provider is recommended.
4. If you are being treated for any health condition, consult your health care provider before beginning this program. It may be wiser to go to a biochemically oriented, residential treatment program where you will have on-site medical supervision and direction during your recovery.
5. If you have a diagnosed mental illness, consider attending a biochemically oriented, residential treatment program where testing and counseling will be individualized and appropriate for you.

## WARNING

Take the Amino Acid Precautions test in Chapter 20. If you are positive for *any* of the conditions, consult your healthcare provider and *do not* do this program without medical guidance.

## IS THIS PROGRAM FOR ME?

Read this entire book and then decide. This program is not difficult, however, it will require your time and attention. You will be taking supplements at nine specific times during the day and preparing nutritious meals and snacks, easy enough once you get used to it. (Consultations with Dr. Suka are available to assist you if needed.)

Your cravings will quickly be reduced or gone in days, when you follow the supplement guidelines. In approximately one week or less you will feel better than you've felt in a long, long time. Is this what you have been searching for?

*Do not attempt to undertake this recovery*
*program without your healthcare provider's*
*knowledge and approval.*

# 18 PROGRAM REQUIREMENTS

Before beginning this program, visit your healthcare provider, who, in all likelihood, won't have a clue about the information you are getting in this book. Sad, but true. If you are able to find a *qualified* integrative healthcare professional, you'll be leagues ahead. Nevertheless, you can request the following tests and follow the guidelines below.

## LABORATORY TESTING

At the minimum, you should have the following tests performed and evaluated by your health care provider to determine your appropriateness for this program.

- CBC (Complete Blood Count)
- CMP (Complete Metabolic Panel)
- TSH, FREE T3, FREE T4 (Thyroid testing)
- AST/ALT (Liver Enzymes)
- Urinalysis

Additional suggested testing:

- DHEA for men and women (Adrenal Steroid)
- PSA for men (Prostate Cancer Antigen)
- Vitamin D 25 Hydroxy

## MEDICATIONS

The recovery program in this book is designed to rebalance your brain chemistry. In order to facilitate that, it's important to follow these guidelines.

- You must be OFF all antidepressants, benzodiazepines, opiates, stimulants, over-the counter pain medications, and all other nonprescription drugs, for your safety and for this program to work well for you.
- Continue Thyroid medication as prescribed by your healthcare provider.
- Continue blood pressure medications but check your blood pressure each morning and evening because it will begin to normalize as you work the program. You will most likely reduce or eliminate the medication entirely. Some amino acids can raise blood pressure. See the AMINO ACID WARNING in Chapter 20.
- Continue any diabetic medications you are on but check your blood sugar level frequently. Your blood sugar levels will begin to normalize the longer you are on the program, and you will likely reduce your medication protocol.
- CAUTION: You should see your healthcare provider before making any medication changes. Do not adjust or discontinue medications on your own.

## SEIZURE PRECAUTIONS

If you have a history of seizures, you must consult your healthcare provider before beginning this program.

## EMERGENCY ASSISTANCE

If you are ever in need of emergency assistance, call 911 immediately.

# PART FOUR

## HOW TO QUIT DRINKING FOR GOOD

# BIOCHEMICAL REPAIR SIMPLIFIED

Before getting into the nitty-gritty of the "how-tos", I want to warn you about your possible reaction to everything you are about to read. There is a lot of information packed into this book. I wrote it as simply as I knew how but you may still become a little overwhelmed as you read it. Two or three re-readings will go a long way to reducing anxiety and clarifying the program.

Have a support person read the book. Discuss the program together. It is not difficult once you have read the instructions a few times. That said, you can always go to www.BrainworksAlcoholRecovery.com and request a consultation. I will be happy to answer your questions and guide you through your recovery program if you want assistance.

OK. Let's get going. As you know by now, alcoholism and other addictions are the result of biochemical imbalances. These imbalances are corrected, not by prescription medications and talk therapy, but by all-natural foods containing the life-giving substances the brain and body must have in order to survive and to become free of all the unnatural physical, emotional, mental and spiritual by-products of addictions.* (See end of chapter.)

The brain and body of an alcohol-dependent person are severely depleted of necessary vitamins, minerals, amino acids, essential fatty acids, enzymes and trace elements. Because undernourished, alcohol-addicted people have difficulty metabolizing food, high levels of supplements are required in order for the body to absorb enough to revitalize itself. Nourishing, healthy foods have to replace the foods that are contributing to the addiction.

All supplements are simply food. Dr. Carl Pfeiffer, founder of the Princeton Bio-Center and pioneer amino acid researcher stated, *"We have found that if a drug can be found to do the job of medical healing, a nutrient can be found to do the same job."*[1]

The following results occur as the brain and body are being biochemically, or naturally, repaired, without the use of prescription medications:

- Absence of craving and tremors
- Elimination of anxiety
- Relief from depression and suicidal thoughts
- Elimination of racing thoughts

- Improved memory and concentration
- Improved sleep
- Recovery from fatigue and exhaustion
- Increased energy and motivation
- Stabilized emotions
- Elimination of aggression, irritability and sudden anger
- Absence of panic attacks
- Reduction or elimination of obsessive-compulsive behaviors
- Reduction of physical pain
- Reduced cholesterol levels
- Normalized blood sugars

*Many emotional and mental symptoms are*
*relieved simply by normalizing brain chemistry.*

Researcher and author Emanuel Cheraskin, MD, states, in reference to addictions, *"Too much therapeutic emphasis has been placed on psychological factors, while more basic biochemical deficiencies and defects in body chemistry have received relatively little attention."*[2]

## MEDICATIONS OR FOOD SUPPLEMENTS?

Although medications are commonly used in addiction recovery programs, they are not successful long term. Prescription medications make the neurotransmitters work harder and longer. They alter brain chemistry for temporary symptom relief, but they don't restore or rebuild the neurotransmitters. These prescriptions actually create further biochemical imbalances, lead to additional addictions, and make profits for the pharmaceutical companies.

Why are alcoholics prescribed benzodiazepines, smokers prescribed nicotine and opiate users prescribed synthetic opiates? Why not just prescribe alcohol for alcoholics? Only the pharmaceutical companies benefit from this legal drug dealing. Have you noticed that it also creates repeat customers? It's time to get real.

Pioneers in the field of orthomolecular, (functional, integrative) medicine have been *successfully* treating patients with mood disorders, mental illness, schizophrenia, and addictions for years. There is a wealth of literature and science most medical physicians have never read and we are the losers because they fail to provide us with the treatment opportunities we deserve.

Only by providing the missing nutrients that are natural to the body, can the neurotransmitters and biochemistry of the entire body be made whole. The substances that repair the biochemistry are amino acids along with their co-factors of vitamins, minerals, essential fatty acids, enzymes and trace elements.** (See end of chapter.) These substances are found naturally from food sources and cannot be patented by pharmaceutical companies, therefore there is no profit in producing them. Only by producing synthetic medications that can be patented, can the pharmaceutical company's profit.

While some of the new drugs being used for addiction recovery help to alleviate the symptoms and speed up the process of detoxification, they also create another addiction that requires a weaning-off process, sometimes more painful than the detoxification from the original substance.

All medications have multiple side-effects. Just listen to television commercials for fad medications. Additional medications, commonly prescribed for these side effects, further alter but do not repair brain chemistry. I have frequently seen hospital patients receiving as many as twenty-four or more *different* medications in a single day. This is not recovery. It's prescription mania.

Consider the adverse effects from taking prescription medications. According to the Federal Agency for Healthcare Research & Quality and The National Academy of Sciences' Institute of Medicine:

- 4.5 million Americans yearly go to their doctor's office or to the emergency room for adverse effects due to prescription medications taken as directed.
- 2 million adverse effects from medications occur with hospital inpatients yearly.
- Prescription medications are the 4th leading cause of hospital DEATHS topped only by heart disease, cancer, and stroke.

*The death rate from prescription drugs is*
*three times greater than from illegal drugs.*[3]

Donald W. Light, a medical sociologist and editor of *The Risks of Prescription Drugs,* a book that reviews current evidence of medication problems, wrote, "There are tens of millions of milder reactions, some of which are quite damaging to people even though they're medically regarded as minor." [4]

*The bottom line is that prescription medications*
*do not restore dysfunctional brain chemistry back to normal.*

*Proof is in the 82% relapse rate.*

On the other hand, all-natural, non-addictive, over-the-counter food supplements, *formulated specifically for biochemical restoration,* combined with *nutrition therapy,* are on the cutting edge of alcohol recovery breakthroughs. The good news is that there are an increasing number of integrative medical physicians who are knowledgeable about the biochemical approach to recovery.

Step One of the 12 Steps states: *"We admitted we were powerless over alcohol."* That statement is absolutely true. Once addicted, the conscious mind is powerless over whatever one is addicted to. The only sure method of recovery is to restore the brain's dysfunctional chemistry to normal using the natural substances the brain and body need for biochemical restoration.

## ARE FOOD SUPPLEMENTS SAFE?

There have never been any deaths attributed to the ingestion of food supplements taken appropriately and there are no adverse side effects from the ingestion of food supplements taken appropriately. What makes the most sense to you?

## FOOD SUPPLEMENTS

The restorative micronutrient and nutritional program suggested in this book has been specifically designed for alcohol detoxification and neurotransmitter restoration and is based upon thirty years of research and actual experience with addictions.

When you purchase your supplements buy the best grade available and look for ingredients that are free from sugar, wheat, starch, yeast, soy, corn, egg, dairy, artificial flavors, colors and preservatives. Capsules, powder, and liquid forms make for the easiest digestion.

You will be taking these supplements frequently throughout the day, before and with meals, between meals, and before bedtime. Your brain needs a constant supply of these substances throughout the day in order for the detoxification and rebalancing of brain chemistry to be as swift and as thorough as possible. You will make the supplement schedule one of your most important items on your daily calendar.

Actually, how long does it take to swallow a few capsules and drink a glass of water? You will also discover how to get rapid relief from opening up capsules and placing the powder directly under your tongue.

The first six to eight weeks is a good beginning. However, your brain may need from twelve to twenty-four months, or more, to become fully restored to normal and, perhaps, become better than it has ever been.

You should continue taking the restoration food supplements for twelve to twenty four months for complete recovery. Some food supplements are encouraged as a daily habit for life, just as they are for everyone, RDS notwithstanding.


## NUTRITION

In this program you will develop sound nutritional habits to support your ongoing recovery. Actually, you'll enjoy eating a huge array of healthy and delicious foods. (If you are overweight, you will probably lose weight. If you are underweight, you will probably gain weight.)

You won't count calories. You will eat as much as you like of healthy foods to restore your brain and body back to health. You won't need to spend lots of time making meals. However, if you enjoy cooking, you'll have an opportunity to be creative, but it isn't necessary.

You will be eating three meals a day with snacks in between meals, but don't let that scare you. Before you begin the program, your brain isn't yet able to even comprehend just how much you will enjoy the nutritional program and how much better you will feel very soon.

Just imagine having increased energy and decreased anxiety and depression. Imagine having a clearer mind and improved memory. Imagine long nights of sound refreshing sleep. Imagine looking forward to life every day.

The nutritional plan is not fanatical. You will not be eating weird, awful tasting food. Healthy, fresh, organically grown, local fruits and vegetables will be the mainstay, along with chicken, turkey and fish for protein, with an occasional bit of beef, if you choose. Of course, junk food will not be on the menu as those "non-foods" are named "relapse". Canned and processed foods are a thing of the past, including processed cheese, luncheon meats, and soft white breads and rolls. But you knew that, didn't you?

Your new nutritional program will become a way of life, a life free of addiction and cravings. It will take time and a little bit of effort in the beginning but I promise you, it will become an easy and enjoyable second nature to you very quickly.


## HYPOGLYCEMIA: SUGAR AND CAFFEINE

Studies show that probably 100% of alcoholics are hypoglycemic (low blood sugar). Because alcohol is sugar to the brain, because most alcoholics crave sugar and eat junk food, because the body can't metabolize "real" food, hypoglycemia (low blood sugar) must be addressed. If not, diabetes will develop. This is a common complication after years of unabated drinking. And, hypoglycemia may be the *leading* cause of relapse! In this program you will find out just how much you have missed good food and will begin to enjoy eating *real* food.

*Sugar is four times more addictive than cocaine.*

Refined sugars, sodas, white foods (bread, rice, pasta, potatoes, French fries, etc.), and sweets are contributing to relapse. In 1968, in a memo to AA's physicians, Bill W. wrote that "we alcoholics try to cure these conditions [of hypoglycemia], first by sweets and then by coffee...In exactly the wrong way, we are trying to treat ourselves for hypoglycemia."[5]

These foods are "sister-foods" to alcohol and are a major cause of craving. It doesn't take long to stop desiring these foods when healthy foods are substituted for sugars. The supplements you will be taking will reduce your desire for them.

Caffeine needs to be eliminated. I can hear some of you now. *"This is just too much."* No. Your alcohol addiction is *too much*. Remember, if you decided to do this program, you also committed to *doing whatever it takes to overcome the alcohol addiction.* Caffeine contributes to hypoglycemia and decreased energy. (It also removes those amino acids from your body.)

Caffeine inhibits the creation of serotonin, the emotional relaxer, and depletes the body of vitamin C, magnesium, calcium, zinc, potassium and the B vitamins. It also hinders the normal metabolism of GABA which explains the increased anxiety people feel after drinking several cups of coffee.

Believing that junk foods and caffeine are *necessities* in your life is just rationalization, an excuse to avoid kicking the addiction. They are not *necessities* and you will quickly realize that for yourself once you are on the program, I promise.

\* Following the recent announcement from American Society of Addiction Medicine (ASAM) that addictions are the result of brain dysfunction, fears were raised that this news will cause the medical community to increase the use of medications in an attempt to repair dysfunctional brain chemistry. We need to educate everyone that prescription medications foster continued addictions and that there already exists thirty years of successful addiction treatment using all-natural nutrient replacement therapy.

\*\* Micronutrients (trace elements) are nutrients required by humans and other living things throughout life in small quantities to orchestrate a whole range of physiological functions, but which the organism itself cannot produce. For humans, they include dietary minerals in amounts generally less than 100 micrograms/ day—as opposed to macro-minerals which are required in larger quantities. The micro-minerals, or trace elements, include at least iron, cobalt, chromium, copper, iodine, manganese, selenium, zinc and molybdenum. Micronutrients also include vitamins, which are organic compounds required as nutrients in tiny amounts by an organism.

# AMINO ACID PRECAUTIONS

Before purchasing your amino acid micronutrients and food supplements, READ these precautions and…

**Please consult a <u>knowledgeable</u> healthcare practitioner before taking ANY amino acids if ANY of the following statements apply to you.**

- You tend to react to supplements, foods or medications with unusual or uncomfortable symptoms.
- You have a serious physical illness, particularly cancer.
- You have severe liver or kidney problems (e.g. Lupis).
- You have an ulcer (amino acids are slightly acidic). [This does not apply if you take all amino acids under the tongue and do not swallow them.] <sup>Insert by Dr. Suka.</sup>
- You are pregnant or nursing (a complete amino blend is usually acceptable, but not individual aminos.)
- You have schizophrenia or other mental illness.
- You have phenylketonuria (PKU).
- You are taking any medications for mood problems, particularly MAO inhibitors or more than one SSRI/SNRI.

Please check off and avoid or be cautious about trying the supplements indicated on the right if you have:

(DL-Phenylalanine = DLPA)

| | | |
|---|---|---|
| High blood pressure | L-Tyrosine or D-Phenylalanine | DLPA |
| Very low blood pressure | GABA | |
| Migraine headaches | L-Tyrosine or D-Phenylalanine | DLPA |
| Bipolar spectrum tendencies* | L-Tyrosine or D-Phenylalanine | DLPA |
| Bipolar spectrum tendencies | L-Glutamine | |
| Severe Depression | Melatonin | |
| Asthma | L-Tryptophan & 5-HTP | Melatonin |
| Overactive thyroid or Hashimoto's | L-Tyrosine or L-Phenylalanine | DLPA |
| Excessively high cortisol output | 5-HTP only | |
| Carcinoid tumor | L-Tryptophan & 5-HTP | |
| Melanoma | L-Tyrosine or D-Phenylalanine | DLPA |
| Lymphatic cancer | L-Glutamine | |

* In approximately 50% of bipolar cases, L-Glutamine can trigger mania. *Note*: L-Glutamine can sometimes relieve bi-polar depression without triggering mania. (SAM-E, St. John's Wort, bright therapeutic lamps, and too much fish or flax oil may also trigger mania.)

**Even if your health care provider agrees that you can try amino acids
(or any other nutrients), if you experience discomfort
of any kind after taking them, stop taking them immediately.**

Name _____ Date _____

© Julia Ross, author of *The Mood Cure* (Penguin 2004) and *The Diet Cure* (Penguin 2012) This information is reprinted with permission of Julia Ross, MA, author of The Diet Cure and The Mood Cure.

# AMINO ACIDS AND WHAT TO PURCHASE

Amino acids are natural proteins, the building blocks of all life. We eat and drink them every day without a second thought. Excess aminos that our body can't use are flushed from our system within four hours. (Alcohol flushes aminos out even before they can be metabolized.) If our neurotransmitter levels are normal, we don't need amino acid supplements. However...

**If neurotransmitter levels are deficient, amino acids
must be present in order to restore neurotransmitter levels to normal.**

Because individuals with an alcohol addiction are low in all four neurotransmitters, you probably need all the amino acids listed.

If you take an amino acid that you don't need, you may have a slight temporary negative reaction. If that occurs, discontinue taking that specific amino acid. Any negative reactions you may have are quickly resolved and are not serious, as long as you are following the Precautions in Chapter 20. Negative reactions mean that you already have enough of that amino and don't need to take it or you have taken the amount you need and don't need to increase the dosage.

Amino acids are precursors to the formation of neurotransmitters and specific aminos follow pathways to creating specific neurotransmitters.

## NEUROTRANSMITTER PATHWAYS

AMINO ACIDS lead to the formation of NEUROTRANSMITTERS

- ➤ L-Tyrosine leads to the formation of Dopamine, then to norepineprhine and epinephrine.
- ➤ L-Tryptophan leads to 5HTP which leads to the formation of Seratonin.
- ➤ GABA is an amino acid that leads to the neurotransmitter GABA.

➢ **D-Phenylalanine (DPA) leads to DL-Phenylalanine (DLPA) which leads to the formation of Endorphins.**

➢ **DL-Phenylalanine (DLPA) also mildly increases Dopamine.**

➢ **L-Glutamine leads to the formation of GABA.**

Some other amino acids perform necessary functions as well and will assist in making your recovery relatively comfortable and symptom-free. The suggested aminos for your recovery are:

- **L-TYROSINE  for Dopamine**
  INCREASES ALERTNESS, ENERGY, MENTAL FOCUS, MEMORY, DRIVE, ENTHUSIASM
- **5HTP for Serotonin**
  POSITIVE OUTLOOK, FLEXIBILITY, EMOTIONAL RELIEF, SELF-CONFIDENCE, SENSE OF HUMOR, HAPPINESS, DEPRESSION RELIEF
- **GABA for GABA**
  CALMNESS, RELAXATION AND STRESS TOLERANCE
- **DLPA  for Endorphins and Dopamine**
  EMOTIONAL & PHYSICAL PAIN RELIEF, PLEASURE, LOVING FEELINGS, COMFORT
- **L-TAURINE**
  CALMING, STABILIZING HEART, BRAIN, & CENTRAL NERVOUS SYSTEM
- **L-THEANINE**
  LOWERS STRESS, ANXIETY, INCREASES MENTAL ACUITY, SUPPORTS HEART AND IMMUNE HEALTH
- **L-GLUTAMINE  for Low Blood Sugar  (Hypoglycemia)**
  STOPS CRAVINGS

## PURCHASING YOUR RECOVERY PROGRAM AMINO ACIDS AND SUPPLEMENTS

Before beginning your recovery program, purchase the following amino acids. I suggest purchasing two bottles of each amino acid to last for the first four weeks, and in some cases longer.

**Buy capsules so you can open them to place the powder directly under your tongue.**

- **L-TYROSINE  500 mg**
- **5HTP 50 mg**
- **GABA 500 mg**
- **DLPA  (DL-Phenylalanine) 500 mg**

- **L-TAURINE 500 mg**
- **L-THEANINE  100 mg**
- **L-GLUTAMINE 500 mg**

## DO NOT SACRIFICE QUALITY FOR COST.

You can purchase the amino acids and the co-factor supplements individually in health-food stores, or on-line. For high quality amino acids, you can order a complete 30-day package of all the recommended amino acids from www.BrainworksAlcoholRecovery.com.

# ***IMPORTANT***

## Buy a blood pressure and pulse monitor for daily measuring and recording.

## MANAGING YOUR SUPPLEMENTS

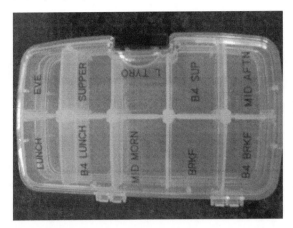

Individuals in our residential treatment program store their supplements in several fishing tackle boxes. One box has ten bins on each side which accommodates two days worth of supplements. We label the bins with the time of day the supplements are to be taken. On each side of the box an extra bin allows for extra L-Glutamine and any other amino you might also want to carry for quick relief.

These boxes are easy to travel with. When you are out for just a few hours at a time, just slip your supplements into a plastic bag and off you go.

*Disclaimer: This information is not a substitute for medical advice from your health care practitioner.*

# CO-FACTORS AND WHAT TO PURCHASE

Vitamins, minerals, essential fatty acids, enzymes and trace minerals are the co-factors that are necessary to metabolize the amino acids. In the past, people didn't think much about supplements because the food they ate was nutritious and supported all their needs. Not so today. Even organic foods are subject to depleted soils, acid rain, airborne chemicals, and polluted water. Animals are raised on grasses that no longer have essential nutrients. Then they are fed corn (genetically modified and lacking nutrients) to fatten them up.

At the end of last July, I drove past fields where they were beginning to pick tomatoes. There was not a single ripe red one anywhere on the vines. Since the nutrients develop only as the fruit or vegetable ripens on the vine, these green beauties had no nutritional value. In addition, the fields have not been allowed to lie fallow, nor have the crops been rotated. (Bacteria in the soil, that feed the plants, multiply only when fields are fallow, or with crop rotation.) Looking pretty, red, and ripe, doesn't mean vine ripened.

In addition to assisting in the metabolism of the amino acids, restoring health and maintaining recovery *requires* food supplementation.

## DO NOT SACRIFICE QUALITY FOR COST

Poorly compounded supplements are immediately flushed from the body with no effect except to deplete your pocketbook.

## SUGGESTED CO-FACTORS FOR ALCOHOL DETOXIFICATION AND REBALANCING OF BRAIN CHEMISTRY

Take these supplemental co-factors daily as suggested for the rest of your life. WHAT DID I JUST READ? Yes, for life. You will eat less, maintain your good health, and avoid relapse. If this shocks you, remember that daily intake of booze is the alternative.

- Vitamin C POWDER (smallest bottle) to take if you have a negative reaction to any amino acid. It will reverse the reaction in minutes. If you have no negative reactions to any amino, just use the powder as part of your daily regimen instead of the tablet. It won't go to waste. (You won't need to buy this again in the future.)
- Vitamin/Mineral Formula appropriate for your age and gender
- Vitamin B6  50 mg (Vitamin B is converted into P-5-P. Scot/Irish people don't absorb B6 very well. For better bioavailability, you can take P-5-P.)
- Vitamin B12 1000 mcg This should be a sublingual, under-the-tongue, tablet.
- Vitamin C 1000 mg Sustained Release
- Vitamin D3 5000 IU minimum.
- Inositol Powder 1000 mg
- Vitamin E 400 IU
- Calcium/Magnesium Complex  1000 mg
- Omega 3 1000 mg (Fish oil or Krill oil is easier to digest than Flax Seed Oil)
- Garlic Kyolic
- Acai Berry 1000 mg
- Turmeric 500 mg (or Meriva® which has more bioavailability) (For heart and liver which are currently stressed.)
- Chromium 200 mcg (Hypoglycemia/Diabetes)
- CoQ-10 60 mg One daily  if you are over 50
- Acidophilus, Bifidophilus, and other probiotics for yeast overgrowth (Candida)
- Valerian Root 500 mg for sleep if needed (optional)

NOTE: When purchasing these supplements check for any ingredients that you may be allergic to, such as: wheat, gluten, soy, milk, eggs, fish, peanut oil, yeast, sugars, colors, preservatives.

Purchase your supplements now so that you will have them ready, along with your amino acids, on the day you begin your recovery program. There are many good quality supplements on the market and many poor to worthless supplements, as well. I suggest two proven quality sources below, however you can do some homework and choose any supplement brand that is of high quality.

## RECOMMENDED SOURCES FOR HIGH QUALITY SUPPLEMENTS

Life Extension: www.lef.org  1-800-678-8989
Bronson Vitamins: www.bronsonvitamins.com  1-800-235-3200

## ORDERING A RECOVERY SUPPLEMENT PACKAGE

You can purchase the amino acids and the co-factor supplements individually in health-food stores, or on-line. For high quality amino acids, you can order a complete 30-day package of all the recommended amino acids from www.BrainworksAlcoholRecovery.com.

*Disclaimer: This information is not a substitute for medical advice from your health care practitioner.*

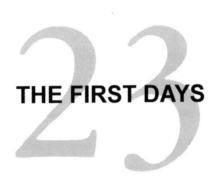

# THE FIRST DAYS

Before actually beginning your recovery program, there are a few things you should do to enhance and protect your recovery.

1. Complete the SYMPTOM CHECKLIST WEEK ONE at the end of this chapter. In order to gauge your progress, I urge you to complete a checklist on Week Three, Week Six, then at Three Months and again at Six Months. It is often difficult to remember how you felt in the past. These Checklists will be powerful motivators for you as you visually watch your progress from week to week and month to month. You will find more checklists later on in this book.
2. Remove all alcohol, including mouthwash, rubbing alcohol and all alcohol containing products, from your living quarters, office, car, and wherever else you have stashed it.
3. Medications used by other members of the family should be locked up and the key kept by your support person. This is for your own protection until your very real cravings and neurotransmitters stop sending you compelling survival messages.
4. All medications no longer prescribed by the participant's physician should be destroyed and all medicine bottles properly disposed of. (This is good advice for everyone.)
5. From now on avoid all drinking parties, bars and drinking buddies. I know this is tough, but if you continue to see drinkers, chances are very good that they will persuade you to drink with them. Really, your best friend, up until now, was the alcohol, not them.

## WHERE TO DETOX

If you have consulted with your healthcare provider and have been given the go-ahead to detox on your own, and if you have stopped drinking in the near past with little or no withdrawal symptoms, and you carefully follow the guidelines below, you may consider doing your detox days at home under the watchful supervision of a non-drinking person.

Alternatively, you may decide to go to a hospital or other medically supervised facility for the first few days of abstinence in order to safely manage your withdrawal symptoms. If you choose to do this, just begin following your recovery protocol and nutritional plan immediately upon returning home.

## BEGINNING THE RECOVERY PROGRAM

1. **Keep drinking** until the evening before you are ready to begin your recovery program, unless you have already stopped drinking.
2. **Decrease** your drinking as much as possible up to that time.
3. **Your last drink** will be the night before the day you begin your recovery program. Don't begin the recovery program until you are ready to stop drinking all alcohol. You can't drink and recover at the same time. You'll be wasting your time and money.
4. **Begin** your recovery program the morning following your last drink the previous night.
5. DO NOT DRIVE. STAY AT HOME AND AVOID STRESSFUL SITUATIONS. Turn off the phone. You are "out of town and unavailable" to the rest of the world for **two or three days.**
6. During the first two to three days of your recovery program, **HAVE ANOTHER PERSON STAY WITH YOU,** *and in your presence,* **AT ALL TIMES.** This will help you to stay motivated and provide emotional support, as well as safety should you need emergency assistance. You may need assistance with your nutrient protocol, as well. After two or three days you should be feeling much better and able to continue with your usual daily activities.

## EMERGENCY ASSISTANCE

If you are in need of emergency assistance call 911 <u>immediately</u>.

**SYMPTOM CHECKLIST WEEK ONE** DATE_____

INSTRUCTIONS: Put a number from **zero** (no symptoms) to **ten** for each symptom you have, with **one being slightly felt or hardly ever felt** and **ten being strongly felt or felt all the time.**

_____ Cravings for alcohol

_____ Uses alcohol regularly

_____ Tendency to allergies, asthma, hay fever, rashes

_____ Bad dreams

_____ No dream recall

_____ Unstable moods, frequent mood swings

_____ Blurred vision

_____ Frequent thirst

_____ Bruises easily

_____ Confusion

_____ Nervous stomach

_____ Poor sleep, insomnia, waking up during the night

_____ Nervous exhaustion

_____ Indecision

_____ Can't work under pressure

_____ Cravings for sweets

_____ Depression

_____ Feelings of suspicion, paranoia

_____ Light-headedness, dizziness

_____ Anxiety

_____ Fearfulness

## SYMPTOM CHECKLIST WEEK ONE continued

_____ Tremors, shakes

_____ Night sweats

_____ Heart palpitations

_____ Compulsive, obsessive, driven

_____ Manic-depressive (cyclical mood changes)

_____ Suicidal thoughts

_____ Irritability, sudden anger

_____ Lack of energy

_____ Magnifies insignificant events

_____ Poor memory

_____ Inability to concentrate

_____ Sleepy after meals or late in the afternoon

_____ Chronic worrier

_____ Difficulty awakening in the morning

TOTAL THE NUMBERS FOR YOUR SCORE: _____

Adapted from *Seven Weeks to Sobriety* by Joan Mathews Larson, PhD

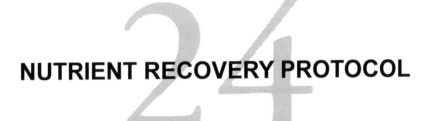

# NUTRIENT RECOVERY PROTOCOL

## AMINO ACID PRECAUTIONS

Carefully read the precautions in Chapter 20 if you have not already done so. DO NOT take any designated amino acids that are contraindicated.

## IMPORTANT – TAKE YOUR VITAL SIGNS

Every day take your blood pressure and check your pulse before taking the aminos in the morning and again before bedtime. Keep a written record of your progress. Most people find they no longer need blood pressure medication after a few days on the program. CAUTION: Do not lower or stop any medication without the advice of your health care provider. Lower the L-Tyrosine if your **blood pressure rises** above your normal.

## HOW TO BEGIN YOUR AMINO ACIDS  (FOR ADULTS ONLY.)

Begin the morning after your last drink. You will begin by trialing your amino acids ½ hour BEFORE breakfast. Don't drink any caffeine or eat anything.

1. **To begin,** you will **trial the aminos, one amino at a time.** Start with 500 mg of L-Tyrosine. Open the capsule and **place the amino powder under your tongue.** Let it dissolve. Don't drink anything. (**Toss the capsule.**) Wait five to fifteen minutes and notice any effects, physical and emotional.
2. If you get a **negative reaction, do not take any more of this amino for a few days.** You can trial it again in three to four days. Do not continue to take any amino that gives you a negative reaction. This is why you trial the amino and the dosage in the beginning. **Do not take more than one capsule at a time until you have completed the trials.**

3. If you get a negative reaction (rare), you will get quick (within minutes) relief by adding 1000 mg of pow-dered Vitamin C to 4 ounces of water. Stir and drink. (Aminos naturally leave the body in one to four hours even without taking the Vitamin C.)

4. Next, trial 500 mg of DLPA (DL-Phenylalanine). Place the powder under your tongue and let it dissolve, without water. Wait five to fifteen minutes and notice any effects, physical and emotional.

5. Next, trial 500 mg of GABA. Place the powder under your tongue in the same manner. Wait five to fifteen minutes and notice any effects, physical and emotional.

6. It isn't necessary to trial the L-Taurine, the L-Theanine, or the L-Glutamine. Just place the lowest dosage of each under your tongue. You can take them all together. Wait 10 minutes and then...

7. Have your breakfast. Begin all of your co-factor supplements with breakfast the first day. Take them during or immediately after your meal to avoid a fishy or other unpleasant taste (rare).

8. In the afternoon you will again trial the 5HTP in the same way starting with a 50 mg capsule. Wait five to fifteen minutes to note the effect.

9. You won't have to do the trials again unless you had a negative effect from any amino. If you did, trial it three or four days later. If you continue to have a negative reaction, just remove that amino from your protocol.

10. In the future place all the amino powders under your tongue that you can easily handle at one time. You may have to divide the amino powders in order to get them to dissolve better. It doesn't matter if the pow-ders get mixed together. They know what to do.

## INCREASING THE DOSAGE

1. From this time forward, begin with the lowest dosage of each amino acid. You can increase the dosage up to the maximum to get more of the relief or result you need. Increase the dosage one capsule at a time and wait one to two days before increasing it again. If your dosage becomes too high, just decrease it the next time you are due to take it.

2. Return to Chapter 21 to remind yourself of the purpose of each amino acid.

3. People usually increase the L-Tyrosine 500 mg every three to four days up to the limit. This amino increases the level of Dopamine that you are deficient in and for which you were taking the alcohol. People with ADD, poor focus or concentration, or low energy and motivation will love this amino for its positive effects.

4. Reduce the L-Tyrosine if the BP level increases. DLPA also increases Dopamine but more gently. It can be substituted for L-Tyrosine. Usually people *lower* their blood pressure medication and come off it because they aren't drinking any more. (Alcohol raises blood pressure.) Don't reduce or eliminate any medication without your healthcare provider's advice.

5. Eat protein and fat at every meal. This will aid in the digestion of your supplements and reduce cravings.

6. Times, such as "mid-morning" and "mid-afternoon", mean half way between your last and next meal on an empty stomach. The exact time of the day isn't so important. However, do not take L-tyrosine or DL-Phenylalanine after mid-afternoon.

7. If you work nights, simply adjust the schedule forward in time to fit your working hours using your meal times as the gauge for when to take the in-between aminos.

8. The protocol is designed to give you a lift in the morning and slowly relax you in the late afternoon and evening, preparing you for a good night's sleep.

9. Use GABA anytime to reduce anxiety or take Inositol as directed.

10. Keep in mind that L-Glutamine is your "anytime" relief for craving "anything". Take it whenever you usu-ally start to get the cravings. Take up to 1500 mg if needed. It's your new healthy "addiction."

# CHANGE YOUR ADDICTION
# BECOME AN AMINO ACID ADDICT
# !!! AAA !!!

IMPORTANT: The aminos and co-factors are needed by your brain in a constant fashion in order for the rebalancing to take place. The most important gift you can give yourself now is to stick to the schedule as much as possible. Your brain needs its fuel on a regular basis in order for you to be released from cravings, anxiety, insomnia, and depression.

When you follow this schedule, you should be feeling better within just a few days and much better within just one week.

## DAILY RECOVERY PROTOCOL

KEY: NT – Neurotransmitter, AM – on arising, B – breakfast, MM – mid morning, L – lunch, MA – mid afternoon, D – dinner, BT – bed time

## CHECK YOUR BLOOD PRESSURE
## BEFORE BREAKFAST AND BEFORE BEDTIME AND RECORD.

## ½ HOUR BEFORE BREAKFAST UNDER TONGUE – NO WATER

L-TYROSINE 500-1500 mg
DL-PHENYLALANINE (DLPA) 500-1500 mg
L-GLUTAMINE 500-1500 mg    In addition, take as needed for cravings.
L-THEONINE 100 mg
L-TAURINE 500 mg

## 10 MINUTES BEFORE BREAKFAST UNDER TONGUE – NO WATER

GABA 500 – 1500 mg

## BREAKFAST   Take with or after meal

Vitamin B6 100 mg
Vitamin C 1000 mg
Vitamin D3 5000 IU
Vitamin E 400 IU
Calcium / Magnesium 1000 mg (May take in divided doses throughout the day)
Omega 3 1000 mg
Garlic Kyolic one tablet
Acai Berry 1000 mg (or other antioxidant)
Turmeric 500 mg
Chromium 200 mcg (Consult healthcare provider if taking insulin. Taking this nutrient may result in a reduction of insulin dosage.)
CoQ-10 60 mg   (One daily if you are over 50)
Vitamin B12 1000 mcg (Under the tongue)

## DAILY RECOVERY PROTOCOL continued

### MID-MORNING UNDER TONGUE – NO WATER

L-TYROSINE 500-1500 mg
DL-PHENYLALANINE (DLPA) 500-1500 mg
L-GLUTAMINE 500-1500 mg    In addition, take as needed for cravings.
L-THEONINE 100 mg
L-TAURINE 500 mg

### 10 MINUTES TO ½ HOUR BEFORE LUNCH UNDER TONGUE – NO WATER

GABA 500 – 1500 mg

### LUNCH   Take with or after meal

Vitamin/Mineral Formula
Vitamin B6 50 mg
Vitamin C 1000 mg
Omega 3 1000 mg
Garlic Kyolic one tablet
Turmeric 500 mg
Chromium 200 mcg

### ANYTIME TO PREVENT ANXIETY OR PANIC - INCREASES GABA LEVELS

Inositol Powder 1000 mg under tongue 1 to 4 times daily as needed.

### MID-AFTERNOON   UNDER TONGUE – NO WATER

5-HTP 50-200 mg
DL-PHENYLALANINE (DLPA) 500-1500 mg by 3 pm
L-GLUTAMINE 500-1500 mg    In addition, take as needed for cravings.
L-THEONINE 100 mg
L-TAURINE 500 mg

### 10 MINUTES TO ½ HOUR BEFORE SUPPER UNDER TONGUE – NO WATER

GABA 500 -1500 mg   May take anytime as needed for anxiety.

### SUPPER   Take with or after meal

Vitamin C 1000 mg
Omega 3 1000 mg
Chromium 200 mcg
Probiotic of your choice

### DAILY RECOVERY PROTOCOL continued

## 1 – 2 HOURS BEFORE BEDTIME   UNDER TONGUE – NO WATER

5-HTP  50-200 mg
GABA  500–1500 mg
L-GLUTAMINE  500-1500 mg
VALERIAN ROOT  500 mg – one or two **with water** for sleep if needed.

## SOME SPECIFIC AMINO ACID GUIDELINES

- SEROTONIN and DOPAMINE are opposites. Taking L-Tryptophan or 5-HTP (for Serotonin) and L-Tyrosine (for Dopamine) **together** will **cancel** each other out. As you will see in the protocol, we want the lift of Dopamine from morning to mid-afternoon and the relaxing effect of Serotonin from mid-afternoon through the evening.
- Because DL-PHENYLALANINE (DLPA) (for Endorphins) also increases Dopamine, take it only in the morning and up to mid-afternoon. For *physical* pain relief *after* mid-afternoon, take D-PHENYLALANINE (DPA).
- SEROTONIN leads to the creation of MELATONIN, the sleep aid. When taking Melatonin by itself fails to induce sleep, it's usually because the Serotonin level is too low. When there is adequate Serotonin, Melatonin will automatically start to develop as daylight fades. To induce sleep, two hours before going to bed, turn lights down low, reduce sounds such as the TV volume, and do things that don't require concentration. This will increase the amount of Melatonin that is being produced in preparation for a good night's sleep. You can also add Valerian Root to induce relaxation and sleep.
- GABA assists Serotonin in regulating Dopamine levels. It can be taken anytime, as needed and in combination with any other amino acids to calm down, chill out, reduce anxiety, and relax. It's also helpful in reducing PTSD symptoms. **(If you have breathing problems after taking GABA, immediately discontinue it. This is rare and has a 1/1000 probability.)**
- L-GLUTAMINE is taken to relieve the symptoms of low blood sugar and whenever you are craving sugar, sweets, and alcohol. This amino does NOT need a trial. It's safe to take whenever it is needed.

## DIGESTION

If you have heartburn after meals, consider taking a digestive enzyme to help digest your food. You can check this out with a homoeopathist or a naturopath.

## TO DO IT OR NOT TO DO IT

David, my husband and a recovery coach, says, "Follow these guidelines precisely and you will greatly increase your odds of a relapse-free recovery." If you are willing and able, but are having difficulties with any part of this alcohol recovery program, you have three good options to keep you on track.

1. You can request telephone consultations with Dr. Suka to answer your questions.
2. You can request a Managed Program with Dr. Suka for an individualized guided *Do-It-Yourself Program*.
3. If you find that you require a more intense one-on-one approach, you can contact Dr. Suka for a list of biochemically-oriented residential treatment programs.

# EAT RIGHT FOR RECOVERY

Probably one of the most important books ever written on the subject of nutrition was *Nutrition and Physical Degeneration* by Weston A. Price, DDS. First published in 1939, republished many times and most lately in 2009, this book is a classic of research, and fascinating reading. (See www.westonaprice.org  for more information) Dr. Price, a dentist and his wife, spent many years visiting the native and aboriginal peoples in every part of the world. He measured and photographed the teeth and jaws of these people while keeping a journal of the foods they ate, their general health, and lifestyle.

These native people had no health diseases, healed quickly from wounds, and had perfect teeth and jaws. They had no jails, no need for police, and lived happy and congenial community lives. There was no obesity, no diabetes, heart disease, cancer, arthritis, or any other of today's common diseases. Yet, when they were exposed to missionaries and traders who gave them white flour, white sugar, jams, refined vegetable oils and canned goods, signs of degeneration quickly became evident. Dental caries, deformed jaw structures, crooked teeth, arthritis and a low immunity to tuberculosis became rampant amongst them. If their children returned to their grandparent's original way of eating before age fourteen, they had none of these deformities or diseases proving that the changes were not genetic, but were due to the changes in nutrition.

Regardless of where these people lived, whether by the sea or inland, in warm or cold climates, anywhere in the world, they had an instinctive ability to eat the foods that would maintain their health. Most importantly, their diets were high in animal protein and natural fats. It made no difference whether the protein and fats came from land animals or fish. They ate an abundance of it.

## WATER, WATER, WATER

Water makes up 70% to 75% of our body. The nervous and all body systems, require enough water to function properly. Water removes toxins and waste from the body. If we aren't drinking enough water, our bodies become stressed and we will have multiple unwanted symptoms. Water in other drinks such as coffee or tea, does not count.

## HOW MUCH WATER SHOULD I DRINK?

Divide your body weight (in pounds) by two. The result is the number of ounces of water you need daily for basic bodily functions. EXAMPLE: Body weight is 150 pounds. Divide that by two. Drink 75 ounces of water daily, or about eight glasses. Some of your water comes from foods and other drinks, such as tea. [Added note: If your physician has placed you on a fluid restriction, follow your physician's orders!]

**Drink filtered or spring water.**
**Begin your day with one to two glasses upon arising.**

## POP AND MOM FOODS –PROTEIN AND FAT

I call protein the POP food and fats the MOM food. We need POP and MOM. POP, or protein, provides us with the amino acids that create our neurotransmitters. MOM, or fats, make up approximately 70% of the brain and are necessary for life. Fats help nutrient absorption, nerve transmission, and maintain cell membrane integrity. Did you know that we don't get fat (overweight) from eating fat? It's sugar and refined flour that makes us fat. *Also, a low fat diet can increase anger and hostility.*

What protein should we eat? Kosher meats, a small amount of red meat if desired, lamb, chicken, turkey and fish, along with plant protein, lentils, and nuts are excellent. *Avoid processed meats.* Because red meat is a storehouse for toxins and hormones, eat only grass fed animal meat. Eggs are an excellent source of protein, as well as dairy products *if* you are not dairy allergic. Vegetarians need to really "beef up" (sorry) their protein from whatever sources that are acceptable to them. No aboriginal tribe was vegetarian.

Healthy fats include butter, yes, real butter. It's wonderful for cooking because it can cook at a high temperature without creating free radicals (molecules that steal away the good nutrients). Coconut oil is also good for cooking. Extra virgin, cold-pressed olive oil is great for salads but not for cooking. Healthy fats are extra virgin olive oil, flax seed oil and fish oil as well as fats from plant sources such as nuts, seeds, avocados, and coconuts. Eat and enjoy.

## FOOD PLAN DIRECTIONS

The following lists are foods you can eat to your heart's content. What was your score for Carbohydrate Addiction (Chapter 7)?

1. **Not positive** for a carbohydrate addiction? Use the **Optimal Health Food Plan.**
2. **Positive** for a carbohydrate addiction? Follow the **Low Carb Food Plan** for at least four weeks before switching to the Optimal Health Food Plan.

# OPTIMAL HEALTH FOOD PLAN

If you are not addicted to carbohydrates, eat these foods and enjoy.

## BEVERAGES

Apricot juice
Carrot juice
Clear broth
Herb teas
Grapefruit
Herb teas
Lemon juice
Lime juice
Loganberry juice
Milk (Limited – See Allergies (Chapter 26)

Orange juice
Pineapple juice
Raspberry juice
Sauerkraut juice
Tangerine juice
Tomato
V-8 juice (not with arthritis)

**(Dilute all fruit juices,
2 parts spring water to 1 part juice)**

## WHOLE GRAINS

Barley
Buckwheat
Millet
Oatmeal
Rice (brown or wild)
Whole wheat

## CHEESES

Cottage cheese
Cream cheese
Gouda, goat, or sheep cheese
Do not use processed cheese, cheese
    spreads, or squeeze-bottle cheese.

## FRUIT (fresh)

Apples
Apricots
Avocado
Banana (limit to 1 daily)
Blueberries
Cantaloupe
Casaba melon
Cherries
Coconut (fresh)
Fruit salad (without grapes)
Grapefruit
Grapes (eat sparingly – high in fructose)
Honeydew melon

Lemon
Lime
Muskmelon
Oranges
Peaches
Pears
Pineapple
Plums
Raspberries
Rhubarb (no sugar added)
Strawberries
Tangerines
Watermelon

## VEGETABLES (fresh)

Artichokes (globe or French)
Asparagus
Beans (green or wax)

Peas (green or edible pod)
Peppers
Pickles (dill or sour)

## OPTIMAL HEALTH FOOD PLAN continued

Beets

Broccoli

Cabbage

Cauliflower

Celery

Cucumbers

Edamame beans

Lettuce

Mushrooms

Olives

Onions (green or raw)

Parsley

Pimentos

Potatoes

Radishes

Rutabaga

Sauerkraut

Soybeans

Spinach

Squash (Hubbard or winter)

Tomatoes

Water chestnuts

Zucchini

## SPROUTS

Alfalfa

Bean

## PROTEIN

Chicken

Turkey

Wild game

Eggs

Fish

Meat (unprocessed) (limit red meat)

Veal

Lamb

Shellfish

## FATS

Butter

Coconut Oil

Extra virgin cold-pressed Olive oil

Avocado

## SALT

Morton's Lite Salt

(half potassium/half sodium)

## RAW NUTS and SEEDS

Almonds

Brazil nuts

Peanuts

Pecans

Pumpkin seeds

Sesame seeds

Sunflower seeds

Walnuts

# OPTIMAL HEALTH FOOD PLAN continued

## LOW CARB FOOD PLAN

If you are addicted to carbohydrates, eat only these foods for four weeks before changing to the Optimal Health Food Plan. Restrict carbohydrates to 50 to 75 grams daily. Dr. Atkins Gram Counter will be helpful with this.

## ANY PROTEINS including:

Beef (unprocessed) (limit red meat)
Chicken
Eggs
Turkey
Veal

Lamb
Fish
Wild game

## RAW NUTS and SEEDS

Almonds
Brazil nuts
Peanuts
Pecans
Pumpkin seeds

Sesame seeds
Sunflower seeds
Walnuts

## VEGETABLES (fresh)

Avocado
Asparagus
Beans (string or wax)
Bean sprouts
Beets
Beet greens
Cabbage
Carrots
Cauliflower
Edamame beans
Eggplant
Kale
Okra
Onions (green or raw)

Peas
Pumpkin
Sauerkraut
Scallions
Spaghetti squash
Spinach
Summer squash
Swiss chard
Tomatoes
Turnips
Water chestnuts
Zucchini

## SAFE FATS

Avocado
Butter
Cream Cheese
Olives
Mayonnaise (no sugar)
Extra virgin cold-pressed Olive oil

Yogurt-plain
Kefir
Buttermilk
Cottage cheese
Coconut oil

## OPTIMAL HEALTH FOOD PLAN continued
### GRAINS
Wasa bread

Soy flour

Crispbread

### FRUIT (fresh) (High in carbs)

Melons

Berries

Grapefruit

### FRUIT JUICES

Water them down to ¼ fruit juice and ¾ water

### GREEN LEAFY LETTUCE / SPINICH

and salad fixings, such as:

Cucumbers

Radishes

Peppers

Herbs

Sprouts

Mushrooms

Olives

Jicama

*Food plans are adapted from Seven Weeks to Sobriety by Joan Mathews-Larson, PhD*

## A WORD (OR TWO) ABOUT GMO'S & BGH

Genetically Modified Organisms (GMO'S) are foods that have had a modified gene inserted into their natural genetic code. Created by Monsanto (the same company that provided chemicals for Agent Orange), these genes are implanted into **corn, soy, sugar beets, cottonseed** and other foods, to create a resistance to their product, Round Up, and other herbicides.

When bugs eat the corn, their bellies explode. Gruesome, but there is more. These modified genes are transferred to cattle and then to human intestines where they continue to multiply and destroy the healthy bacteria in human intestines, creating a "leaky gut syndrome". This allows poisons to enter the blood stream while preventing healthy nutrients from moving into the blood stream.

Some of the symptoms linked to the ingestion of GMO modified foods are:

- Asthma
- Autism
- Cancer
- Infertility
- Decreased Immune System

- Leaky Gut
- Organ Damage
- Spontaneous Abortions
- Tissue Damage

BGH, or Bovine Growth Hormone, is given to cows to increase their milk production and is linked to an increased cancer risk.

## JUST SAY "NO" TO GMO AND BGH

Be aware that genetically modified corn and sugar beets form most of the sweetening in all processed foods. Soy products are not safe, either, being genetically modified, as well.

## BASIC TIPS FOR RELAPSE-FREE RECOVERY

- AMINO ACID ADDICT: Become one.
- DRINK SPRING OR FILTERED WATER ALL DAY LONG.
- EAT BREAKFAST. It prevents obesity and alcohol relapse!
- EAT three meals daily. Small balanced meals with plenty of protein, healthy fats, fresh vegetables and fruit.
- EAT SLOWLY: Put silverware down between bites.
- PORTIONS: A portion is the size of your palm. Use small plates.
- SNACKS: Eat high protein, high fat snacks between every meal.
- POOP: Healthy poop floats. Check it out.
- URINE: Will be straw color or yellow when taking lots of Vitamin B's.
- SLEEP: Get seven to nine hours sleep every night.
- WALK or EXERCISE daily.
- PLAY, have FUN, LAUGH. Don't take things too seriously.
- HUG, KISS, AND LOVE A LOT.

# CANDIDA AND ALLERGY REPAIR

Now that you've taken the Candida and Allergy tests you already have an idea of whether you are allergic to any foods or if you may have Candida. Let's deal with Candida first.

## CANDIDA SYMPTOMS

- Depression
- Disoriented, spacey, light-headed
- Poor memory
- Difficulty concentrating
- Difficulty making decisions
- Bloating, distension, or gas
- Abdominal pain
- Loss of sexual interest or ability
- Vaginal burning, itching, or discharge
- Premenstrual tension or cramps
- Cold hands or feet or physical chilliness
- Pain or swelling in joints
- Chronic eczema, rashes, or itching (anal, under breasts)
- Body odor or bad breath not relieved by washing/brushing
- Chronic sore throat, laryngitis, cough, or tender glands
- Urinary frequency, burning, or urgency
- Pain or tightness in chest, wheezing, or shortness of breath
- Recurrent ear infections, fluid in ears
- Chronic sinus infections
- Food sensitivity or intolerance
- Persistent yeast infections

- Prostatitis, vaginitis, or other reproductive problems
- Frequently exposed to high-mold environments
- Have a sensitivity to mold
- Severe athlete's foot, nail or skin fungus, ringworm, or other chronic fungus
- Treated for internal parasites
- Crave or consume lots of sweets
- Crave or consume lots of starches such as pasta or bread
- Crave or consume lots of alcoholic beverages

**Antibiotics and other drugs as co-factors**

- Taken tetracycline or other antibiotics for one month or longer
- Frequent short courses or other broad-spectrum antibiotics
- Taken prednisone or other cortisone-type drugs for one month or more
- Taken birth control pills for more than a year

If your test results indicate that you have Candida, follow the LOW CARB FOOD PLAN. You will be eliminating the sugars and starches that feed the Candida. Remain on this food plan for at least a month. Of course, you now know that reintroducing sugars into your food plan is a call for Candida to redevelop.

If the Candida persists while you are on this food plan, consult with your health care provider. Diflucan is a prescription drug that can be very helpful in speeding up your recovery. There are many good medications, some of which do work better than natural sources. Using medications with good judgment, and as minimally as possible, is wise. Homeopathy treatment can be very effective, as well.


## ALLERGIES

Allergies can affect your digestive system, skin, respiratory system, muscular system, and more. The most severe allergic reaction is anaphylaxis, which affects many body systems and can be fatal.

The most common allergies are to wheat and dairy products. Allergies to milk and milk products can create severe behavioral and even criminal behaviors. The book *Food and Behavior* by Barbara Reed Stitt, PhD, is an eye-opener. As a Probation Officer, she worked with thousands of adults and school children. When they changed their diets, and removed the offending foods, their criminal behaviors stopped entirely and they became well-adjusted law-abiding citizens. Consider the impact this has on raising children who are difficult to manage. (Her book is available at www.BrainworksRecovery.com.)


## IF YOUR ALLERGY TEST WAS POSITIVE

Ask yourself some questions. Can I easily give up this food? Am I reluctant to give it up? Do I eat it every day? Does it give me pleasure to eat it? If you eat something every day, even several times a day, and don't want to give it up, you are most likely allergic to it. You may not be aware that the symptoms you are experiencing, such as arthritic or muscular pains, runny nose, rashes, depression, irritability and dozens of other symptoms are the result of an allergic reaction to this food that you so dearly love. ("Dearly loving it" is a clue!)


## ELIMINATION DIET

The most effective method for determining if you are allergic to a food is the Home Testing Elimination Diet. This method is even more accurate than any blood or skin test. Here's how to do it.

## DAY 1 TO 5 – ELIMINATION

Stop consuming all the foods you have decided to test. For cravings, take your aminos according to your needs. (Become an Amino Acid Addict.) If you are allergic to any of the foods you are testing, you should start feeling better by day five.

## DAY 5 – THE CHALLENGE

1. Notice if any of your bothersome symptoms have gone away and make a written note of it.
2. On DAY FIVE eat a regular serving of ONE TEST FOOD ONLY for breakfast and again at lunch. Eat nothing else besides that product (an all dairy meal or wheat-only meal, for example).
3. Write down how you feel. Also note your oral temperature, any food cravings, your mood, energy, digestion, respiratory symptoms, bowel function, appetite, skin changes, headaches, sleep patterns and any and all information that your body tells you. You may have a very strong reaction, such as a migraine if you're prone to them. If you get only a little tired, bloated, or headachy after your challenge meals, don't ignore it. If you gain weight or start craving foods again, don't be surprised. It's very helpful to have someone with you when you test your food to observe reactions that you may not be aware of.
4. If you are testing grains for a gluten allergy, test wheat first as it contains the most gluten.
5. Do not eat any more of the food or food group for the next three days.
6. After waiting 72 hours, you can test another food group, milk for instance.
7. Don't eat any foods you have tested until you have finished testing all of the foods you have stopped.
8. Take DLPA or DPA to manage your side effects. (Chapter 21.)
9. If you have a negative reaction, you'll know what food or food group to avoid. If you accidentally eat the food and have a reaction, take two tablets of Alka Seltzer Gold to get rid of it quickly.

## HELPFUL HINTS

1) Keep a detailed food-mood log to monitor your reactions
2) Reintroduce only one food group at a time.
3) Wait two full days before testing another food.
4) Be aware of ALL adverse reactions, no matter how small.
5) Women should test after their period and before PMS.

Delayed reactions, up to 48 hours, can occur so continue to monitor your reactions and write them down, no matter how small or unusual they may appear.

Some people have more severe intestinal problems which can take several months before the intestines can heal. If this testing is not sufficient, I refer you to *The Diet Cure* by Julia Ross, MA, for more detailed guidelines.

# ALLERGY PROGRAM FOOD PLAN

Using this food plan, which automatically **eliminates** both **wheat** and **dairy** products, will make it easier to plan your meals.

## BEVERAGES

Apricot juice

Carrot juice

Clear broth

Herb teas

Lemon juice

Lime juice

Loganberry juice

Orange juice

Pineapple juice

Raspberry juice

Sauerkraut juice

Tangerine juice

V-8 juice (not with arthritis)

**(Dilute all fruit juices, 2 parts spring water to 1 part juice)**

## FRUIT (fresh)

Apples

Apricots

Avocado

Blueberries

Cantaloupe

Casaba melon

Cherries

Coconut (fresh)

Fruit salad (without grapes)

Grapefruit

Honeydew melon

Lemon

Lime

Muskmelon

Oranges

Peaches

Pears

Pineapple

Plums

Raspberries

Rhubarb (no sugar added)

Strawberries

Tangerines

Watermelon

## NUTS and SEEDS

Almonds

Brazil nuts

Peanuts

Pecans

Pumpkin seeds

Sesame seeds

Sunflower seeds

Walnuts

## PROTEIN

Chicken and other fowl

Eggs

Fish

Meat (unprocessed) (limit red meat)

Shellfish

# ALLERGY PROGRAM FOOD PLAN continued

## VEGETABLES (fresh)

Artichokes (globe or French)

Asparagus

Beans (green or wax)

Beets

Broccoli

Cabbage

Cauliflower

Celery

Cucumbers

Lettuce

Mushrooms

Olives

Onions (green or raw)

Parsley

Peas (green or edible pod)

Peppers

Pickles (dill or sour)

Pimentos

Radishes

Rutabaga

Sauerkraut

Soybeans

Spinach

Squash (Hubbard or winter)

Tomatoes

Water chestnuts

Zucchini

## SPROUTS

Alfalfa

Bean

## WHOLE GRAINS

Quinoa

Amaranth

Oats

Rice (brown or wild)

## FATS

Extra virgin cold-pressed Olive oil

Coconut oil

Avacodo

*Food plan is adapted from Seven Weeks to Sobriety by Joan Mathews-Larson, PhD*

## WHAT'S THE FUTURE FOR THE ALLERGY PRODUCING FOODS YOU LOVE?

Remain free of the offending foods for six months. Then, one at a time, you can reintroduce them. Eat the offending food no more than once every four to five days. If you have several offending foods, alternate them so that you are eating only one of them a day.

As you begin to feel like a new person, you will agree that the effort was well worth it.

# 27

## NICOTINE ADDICTION

*Is giving up tobacco a stumbling block for you?*
*Smoking, or chewing, and relapse are twins.*

RON, a divorced, 36 year old father of two sons, came to our residential program chewing 1 to 1&1/2 cans of tobacco daily. He knew we would expect him to stop chewing but we didn't focus on it early in the program.

As a result of taking the aminos and supplements, and eating well, plus the exercise schedule he was on, he found that he had used only two and a half tins in the first two weeks of his 30 day program, without any direction from us.

The third week I asked him to stop chewing and see how he felt. Ron took the L-Glutamine whenever he would usually chew and found he had no more cravings. From that day onward, he didn't chew again and when he left the program after 30 days, he felt he could leave tobacco alone for good. If he felt the desire to chew, he was prepared to take the L-Glutamine, and use some other techniques he had learned (Meridian Tapping – Chapter 29) to remain tobacco free.

When Ron entered the recovery program, his blood pressure was above normal even though he had been taking blood pressure medication for the past four years while drinking heavily at the same time.

We adjusted his recovery protocol hoping to lower his blood pressure and it was coming down, however, it continued to remain above normal for the first two weeks as he continued to chew, even the small amount. When Ron stopped chewing, his blood pressure normalized for the first time in years and remained normal without blood pressure medication.

Ron was eager and highly motivated to continue his recovery program when he returned home and is now well on his way to a relapse-free life.

## TOBACCO

Over 430,000 deaths each year are caused by tobacco, according to the US Department of Health. More than 70 percent of smokers want to stop while fewer than 10 percent succeed. Nicotine addiction is said to be the most difficult addiction to let go of. But then, you knew that, didn't you?

Nicotine is one of the most powerful poisons known. It's so toxic that as few as two or three drops of pure nicotine applied directly to the skin of an average person will kill him or her within minutes. Over 100 different toxins have been found in cigarette smoke. Whether chewing or smoking, nicotine addiction works in the same areas of the brain as other addictive drugs. Nicotine can also make the brain more sensitive to the effects of other addicting drugs, an effect that can last for some time after nicotine exposure.[1]

Another area of research reveals that a common byproduct of smoking is acetaldehyde, the same compound formed when alcohol is metabolized. Just as with alcohol, acetaldehyde combines with endorphins to form compounds that activate GABA and morphine receptors. This gives a feeling of relaxation and, sometimes, euphoria (from dopamine stimulation). Apparently, this is a major factor in the development of smoking addiction.[2]

One currently popular brand of cigarettes proudly advertises that some of their tobacco is cured in whiskey barrels for over a year before being put into cigarettes. Furthermore, all tobacco is cured in sugar. Hypoglycemics, beware. Could this be a cause of craving?

Cigarette paper contains the metal, cadmium, to keep it white. Tobacco smoking is the most important single source of cadmium exposure in the general population. It has been estimated that about 10% of the cadmium content of a cigarette is inhaled through smoking. As much as 50% of the cadmium inhaled via cigarette smoke may be absorbed. On average, smokers have 4–5 times higher blood cadmium concentrations and 2–3 times higher kidney cadmium concentrations than non-smokers.

Despite the high cadmium content in cigarette smoke, there seems to be little exposure to cadmium from passive smoking. Cadmium exposure is a risk factor associated with early atherosclerosis and hypertension, and both can lead to cardiovascular disease.[3]

We are already aware of the complications of lung disease and smoking-induced cancer. Addiction is addiction, regardless of the substance. The whole goal of addiction recovery is to alleviate the *need* for *all* addictive substances. Continuing to smoke or chew tobacco is not recovery.

Many treatment programs allow patients to continue to smoke while in recovery. In some treatment programs where I worked, smoking and chewing were prohibited, and in others it was limited to 12 cigarettes spaced throughout the day. Nicotine addiction is so powerful that when smoking was denied, patients often responded with childish tantrums, threats to the staff, slamming of doors, screaming tirades, and cursing demands to be released from the program.

Experience, using the biochemical restoration model of recovery, has proven that those individuals who do *not* stop smoking will usually relapse on alcohol. What's the point of going through a recovery program if we aren't willing to recover?

We do not accept individuals into our residential program if they are unwilling to give up their nicotine addiction. That's because we want a relapse-free recovery for all of our residents. If they continue to use tobacco, their brain chemistry will remain imbalanced and in survival mode. This will eventually draw them back to alcohol because alcohol will meet their survival needs better than tobacco, alone. However, giving up tobacco is not as difficult as you might think when you have assistance in detoxifying your body and your brain chemistry is being naturally restored.

## HOW TO STOP SMOKING OR CHEWING

Attempting to stop an alcohol addiction and a smoking addiction at the same time is a program headed for disaster. At the **beginning of the third week** on your alcohol recovery program, start the program outlined below. By then your brain is starting to restore biochemical balance.

Millions of ex-smokers have quit. You can too. Here's how to stop smoking.

1.  Set a target date to quit two weeks from today.

2. Continue to eat your healthy food plan. Eat protein and fats (nuts, cheese, meat, eggs, etc.) as snacks to prevent craving.

3. Take L-Glutamine 500 – 1500 mg to prevent or stop cravings. Carry it with you at all times and remember to use it.

4. Maintain your exercise program. It will help counteract any weight gain when you stop smoking.

5. Over the two weeks leading up to your quit date, cut down on cigarettes. This is easier if you take sodium/potassium bicarbonate (Alka-Seltzer Gold) to alkalize your system and reduce your nicotine cravings. Take two tablets every four hours, but no more than eight tablets in any twenty-four hour period.

6. Avoid red meats, cranberries, plums, and prunes (they promote the acidity you are trying to neutralize with the Alka-Seltzer Gold).

7. Drink at least eight glasses of water a day.

8. Avoid nicotine patches because they deliver nicotine even in your sleep.

9. Nicorette gum may be useful.

## *YOU CAN DO IT!!*
## *YOUR ALCOHOL RECOVERY DEPENDS ON IT.*

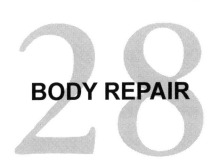

# BODY REPAIR

## FLUSH THE LYMPHATIC SYSTEM

The lymph system is a separate set of vessels running throughout the body. It's responsible for clearing the debris. It contains toxin-filled water, dead cells, dead microorganisms, cellular waste, etc. Whenever this system becomes clogged, the body will become a miserable place to inhabit! Everything becomes stagnant. The body loses its ability to clean itself up.

To see how badly your body is congested, try rubbing the large pocket of lymph nodes located just under and in front of the armpits. If the system is congested, these areas are almost always tender when rubbed. Other areas that may be tender are at the groin and along the spinal column.

Fortunately, for most people, it is relatively easy to open the system up!

1.  **Rub** the areas that are sore once or twice daily. Rub them deeply enough to feel some discomfort, but it is not necessary to create a torturous situation!
2.  **Drink** the prescribed amount of water for the bodily needs. (Remember: take the body weight in pounds, divide by two. The answer is the correct MINIMAL amount of fresh, filtered water in ounces that that body needs for the basic bodily functions.)
3.  **Move** the muscles. The lymph system has no natural pump. It relies upon muscular movement to keep it flowing. Since the leg muscles are the largest muscles in the body, walking or using a rebounder are the exercises of choice.
4.  **Relaxation** is one way to allow the body to put its full attention upon detoxifying. Through adequate sleep and time spent in meditation, or at least sitting still for awhile each day, the body is able to hasten its repair.
5.  **Exercise** increases blood flow, builds muscle tissue, moves the lymph fluids, builds overall stamina, increases self-esteem and creates a sense of self-control and feeling good. It also enables the body to function in a more efficient manner overall.[1]

## MOVEMENT AND STRETCHES

Begin your day with whole-body stretches, standing, bending, and lying on the floor. In particular, focus on moving, stretching, and bending your spine from the neck to the pelvis. Keeping the spine flexible is of the utmost importance for the nervous system. Spend about fifteen minutes awakening your body and preparing it for the day. You will feel energized and improve your ability to focus your thinking, as well.

## INFRA-RED, DRY-HEAT SAUNAS

When alcohol, and other substances, are being metabolized, toxins and residues that are not excreted or eliminated move into the fatty tissues and remain there, sometimes for life. When you are under high stress, from any source, some of these metabolites may be released into your blood stream.

Suddenly, the parts of the primitive brain that house memories of drinking alcohol, and the emotional content of those experiences (the hippocampus and amygdala), signal the reward pathway that a dopamine fix is needed and sudden, unexpected, intense cravings occur as a response. This can happen weeks, months, even years after all drinking has ceased. This is when the person says, *"I don't know what happened. I just drank"*.

So, we want to remove those metabolites, as well as all the accumulated toxins that have been stored in the body for years. Those toxins are contributing to poor health, as well.

The first step is to take infra-red dry-heat saunas five days a week for the first four weeks of recovery. After that, depending upon how much fat you are carrying, you can reduce the saunas to two or three times weekly and then to twice a month for several months.

Steam saunas are too hot for recovering. Those who have been drinking for years usually have increased blood pressure and steam saunas are too hard on the heart. Staying in the dry-heat infra-red sauna for about ten minutes is sufficient. Of course, if you feel your heart pounding or uncomfortable, get out immediately.

Our residential clients have full access to the facilities of a local YMCA that provides these saunas, along with exercise equipment and a swimming pool.

## MASSAGE

I urge you to get weekly full body, one-hour massages for the first four to six weeks, as least. Massage is extremely helpful for removing stress and tension from the muscles, and the removal of toxins from the lymph glands. Emotional blocks are released during these sessions, as well.

The benefits from these sessions include: improved sleep, more energy, relaxation, a sense of well-being, and many other benefits. Plus, we must not ignore the very real benefit of learning to let go of defensiveness while accepting the gift of healing and caring from another.

## AURICULOTHERAPY

Auriculotherapy is acupuncture performed on the ear. The National Acupuncture Detoxification Association has, very successfully, used ear acupuncture since 1985 to help thousands of individuals withdraw and detoxify from addictive substances. This can be a very helpful addition to one's recovery program.

Auriculotherapy can be done quickly. Patients do not have to remove any clothing. Ear acupuncture treatments use needles, but they can be modified for use with needleless methods, such as an electro-stimulation device, magnets, or ear seeds (which can be applied and remain on the ear for several days for continual treatment).

## EXERCISE IS A MUST FOR RECOVERY

Exercise is absolutely necessary for a relapse-free recovery. Your brain and body chemistry depend upon it. Create an exercise plan that you can enjoy and do, for at least forty minutes, four to five days a week. The easiest and totally effective exercise is simply to walk, just fast enough to keep the heart rate up. Experience has proven that walking can often improve mood and relieve depression. Any form of full-body exercise that you enjoy is acceptable. Your health will improve quickly with exercise.

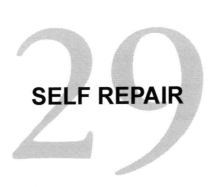

# SELF REPAIR

*"Who am I? Who is the person I've become? I'm a slave to thoughts and emotions I don't like or want. I'm fighting to keep things under control. I'm pretending to be normal. I'm hiding my addiction, trying to keep it a secret, even from myself. The stress is overwhelming. I smile. I try to keep my work up to par. It gets harder and harder every day but I know I'm slipping. Thoughts of drinking fill my mind, even more than thoughts about work or my family. I'm worried about people finding out. I might lose everything. I feel guilty and ashamed. I'm trapped. I'm alone. Where is this going to end up? I'm scared. I'm in a box and I don't know how to get out."*

These are thoughts Michael expressed when we talked. His questions and thoughts were valid. Michael was a highly functioning business executive. His wife was a grade school teacher and they had two young sons. Michael and his wife owned a nice home in a suburban neighborhood, played golf at the country club, and liked to attend cultural events. They socialized frequently with a wide network of social and professional friends, but underneath the façade, Michael was losing himself and his life, and he knew it. Michael was a perfect candidate for this recovery program. He is no longer an alcoholic.

*"I drink four or five glasses of wine every evening, starting about 4:30 in the afternoon. I love my job but it's getting to be too much. They cut down the staff and want the rest of us to take on the extra work load. I feel so responsible to get it all done. I'm a perfectionist and I worry a lot, so the wine helps me to relax. My husband thinks I should quit. I know I'm irritable and moody. I'm not fun to be with any more. I can't sleep at night and I don't have any energy. I used to be so healthy and active. I've actually had panic attacks at work and once I blacked out. That was scary. I think I need to stop drinking but I don't know how. Can you help me?"*

Michele and her husband were both college professors in their fifties. They had no children. They owned a home near the college and another vacation home in the mountains where they frequently spent their weekends hiking and biking together. However, Michele was not enjoying life much anymore. To make up for it, at home she kept busy, constantly cleaning, gardening, repairing, painting, fixing up, rearranging, accomplishing little but keeping active. Drinking allowed her to slow down and forget the racing thoughts in her head.

This wasn't the life she had looked forward to when she graduated from college. She knew she had missed a promotion she really wanted at work due to her inability to concentrate, and her mood swings were causing some concern with her colleagues. Michele appeared sad and lost when she asked for help. She followed the recovery program and successfully regained the life she had lost through drinking.

*RDS creates addiction to alcohol.*
*Alcohol messes with the mind.*

The entire brain is affected by alcohol and other addictive substances. The brain no longer operates fully, and sometimes not even appropriately. Let's look at five brain systems that affect everything in our life. [1]

## LIMBIC SYSTEM

The deep limbic system, at the center of the brain, where the Reward Pathway is located, is the bonding and mood control center. It's essential that we are able to bond with one another. When this part of the brain is imbalanced, people struggle with moodiness and negativity. Distancing from others creates loneliness and reduced self esteem.

## BASIL GANGLIA

These are large structures deep within the brain that control the body's idling speed. When this part of the brain overworks, anxiety, panic, fearfulness, and conflict-avoidance are often the result.

## PREFRONTAL CORTEX

The prefrontal cortex lies at the front tip of the brain. It is the supervisor, helping to stay focused, make plans, control impulses, and make good (or bad) decisions. When this part of the brain is not functioning properly, people have significant problems with attention span, focus, organization, and follow-through.

## CINGULATE

This part of the brain runs longitudinally through the middle part of the frontal lobes. When it is overactive, people have problems getting stuck in certain loops of thoughts, or behavior. Overstimulation of this part of the brain creates repetitive worries, rigidity, and "over-focused" behavior.

## TEMPORAL LOBES

The temporal lobes are located underneath the temples and behind the eyes. They are involved with memory, understanding language, facial recognition, and temper control. When there are problems in these areas, especially the left temporal lobe, people have more temper flare-ups, rapid mood shifts, memory and learning problems.

Dysfunctional brain chemistry affects all areas of the brain, so it's not surprising to experience the down-side of these brain activities. Historically, we have tended to blame people for their misbehaviors and less than socially-acceptable conduct when, in fact, these people are the victims of brains gone haywire.

We are not seeing the *real* person. We are seeing and experiencing a life that is damned up inside a physical brain that isn't fully functioning. This is not mental illness. It's brain sickness.

Fortunately, with the gains in neuroscience, and thirty years of recovery experience, these people can be released from the consequences of their addiction and become whole again.

Sometimes people have a mental or personality disorder before they developed a drinking addiction. Some people have been so damaged by their early life experiences that alcohol was, at first, a relief and a place to hide. I once had a co-worker who saw life as just one bad experience after another. She was so adroit at rapidly turning the best into the worst that she could engage another person for hours with complaints if one let her. Alcohol intensifies, but doesn't cause, these behaviors. As these people recover from alcoholism, they need to address their emotional and mental issues, as well.

Most alcoholics are intelligent, fun, good, caring, enjoyable people who are skilled and successful even as alcohol begins to take over their life. Indeed, many alcoholics remain great friends, and good people to work with and be around, for a long time before the effects of alcohol begin to take their toll on life.

We all know the devastation that alcohol addiction can cause, from health issues, financial crisis, career loss, family disruption, divorce, homelessness, to suicide. There is no reason for anyone to ever go that route again. This is the message we need to send everyone.

There is no shame or blame in this disease. When you discover you are becoming or are addicted to alcohol, *immediately* get the help that will turn your life around.

There are many ways to deal with emotional and behavioral issues that have developed as a result of alcoholism *but* these very good resources won't have much effect if the brain is not biochemically restored.

Consider this analogy. You are a driver-education teacher, and a skilled race car driver to boot. No matter your abilities, if your car is out of gas, has no oil in the crankcase, no water in the radiator, and has flat tires, you're not going anywhere.

The brain needs its fuel in order for you to operate through it at your highest capability. Fix the car, fix the brain, and both can operate efficiently.

Once your initial detoxification is completed and your brain restoration program is in force, these additional resources will get you going again.

## COUNSELING

Counseling is highly recommended as long as the counselor understands the *real* cause of addiction. Any counseling that encourages the belief that you are responsible for your addiction should be avoided. However, wait four to six weeks before beginning counseling, if you need it. Be good to yourself and give your brain time to think clearly again.

Perhaps your social skills have deteriorated. Marriage and family counseling can be very beneficial as long as you are willing to make changes in your behaviors, beliefs, and attitudes and you are not defensive about your past.

## NERUOLINGUISTICS

A Neuro-Linguistics Practitioner can skillfully help you to release the past, and move forward very quickly without being re-traumatized. You won't be asked why you ever did anything. You will be skillfully guided to recreate the new future that you desire.

## MERIDIAN TAPPING

Also known as Emotional Freedom Techniques, (EFT), this is the fastest growing Energy Psychology in the world. It's so powerful that it is now being successfully used with veterans suffering from PTSD (Post Traumatic Stress Disorder).

Dr. Joseph Mercola states *"Without a doubt meridian tapping techniques are the single most consistent and effective intervention in improving one's health that I have ever witnessed in over three decades of studying health."*[2]

Meridian Tapping consists of tapping on specific acupuncture sites around the upper chest and head while repeating phrases or while simply talking about emotional subjects. Very quickly, the emotional "charge" surrounding the issue is released. Layers upon layers of inner blockages are comfortably released in a very short time. You can learn about this technique by going to the web site www.EFTuniverse.com.

There are many alternative therapies that can enhance your healing process. While each one can be very helpful, it's just not practical, nor is it cost or time effective, to do everything. I only mention them in case you have the ability to add one or two to your recovery program. Perhaps you may decide at a later time to try some of these when you have gotten beyond the initial weeks of recovery.

## SOME OTHER SUGGESTED ALTERNATIVE THERAPIES

(There are too many to list them all.)

REIKI   YOGA   TAI CHI   QIGONG   FENG SHUI

DRUMMING   BIOFEEDBACK   HOMEOPATHY   REFLEXOLOGY

ACUPUNCTURE   NATUROPATHIC   MUSIC THERAPY

AROMA THERAPY   ENERGY HEALING   QUANTUM TOUCH®

THERAPEUTIC TOUCH   CRANIAL-SACRAL THERAPY

BRAIN STATE CONDITIONING   CHIROPRACTIC ADJUSTMENT

MYOFASCIAL TRIGGER POINT THERAPY

Regardless of how you choose to address the emotional and behavioral aspects of your recovery, your brain and body repair must come first. You can continue your life-driving education once your vehicles, your brain and body, are restored to working condition.

Be patient. Respect your brain and body. They know what to do when given the proper ingredients to work with. Take some deep breaths, smile, and know you are on your way to a healthier life.

## CHANGE HABITS / CHANGE FRIENDS

The old habits and friends had one purpose; to keep you drinking, to support your drinking, and to keep you deluded about the seriousness and consequences of your drinking. That's powerful and that, alone, WILL drive you back to drinking.

If these habits and friends are allowed to continue influencing your life, your addicted brain chemistry will latch onto them and destroy everything you want to achieve, including your health, your relationships, your job or career, your sanity, and eventually, your life.

If you are reading this book for yourself, or for another, it's imperative to recognize that changing habits and friends is just as important as all the other steps in this book, combined!  That's one of the purposes of AA – to get addicts going to a meeting instead of a bar or liquor store, and to meet other recovering people who will support them instead of encouraging them to drink.

Changing habits *right now* is major. After your recovery is more solidly in place, you will be able to handle some of these situations more effectively, but now, in the beginning, be *compulsive* about avoiding these traps.

## Changing habits means:

1. Getting everything that reminds you of drinking out of your house, office, car, garage, and anywhere else you are storing it, including wine and liquor glasses, decanters, etc.
2. Hide, give away, or destroy pictures of you and your drinking pals.
3. Avoid restaurants where liquor is served
4. Stay away from the beverage area in grocery stores.
5. Fill your non-drinking time with new activities: join a support group, take a self-improvement class, walk, golf, bowl, fish, bicycle, read at a library, join a Meet-Up, volunteer, attend a church group, sing in a choir, do something with carpentry, garden, get a pet, or any activity that inspires you and you enjoy doing it.
6. Be busy. Leisure time without something stimulating to challenge you is a call for alcohol.
7. Take your L-Glutamine before your usual drinking times and when you crave, if you are still craving.
8. Avoid stress by avoiding people who are drama-driven.
9. For anxiety, take your anxiety aminos – GABA, L-Glutamine, and the vitamin, Inositol.
10. Avoid lengthy telephone calls.
11. Stay away from parties, fairs, or celebrations where drinking is prominent including weddings – a great place to fall off the wagon without a second thought!  The bride and groom's marriage won't be ruined because you weren't there. Go to a movie, instead, or invite non-drinking friends to celebrate the newlyweds at your private party while the real one is going on. Be creative and be clean.
12. Avoid TV shows that include drinking or overly emotional scenes. Your own emotions are easily stimulated and can cause you to reach for the bottle before you are even aware of it.
13. Subscribe to the *Good News Network* on the internet.
14. Avoid switching to marijuana, or other substance (including relationships) to create a cross addiction. They will lead you back to alcohol over time.
15. The tobacco habit maintains unbalanced brain chemistry and will return you back to alcohol eventually. You can depend on it. Use your aminos and other supplements to help you quit smoking or chewing.
16. Don't make any major decisions early in your recovery because you still don't have all the mental faculties to think clearly. Sorry, but it's true.

## Changing friends means:

1. Stay away from family members or old friends who attempt to sabotage your recovery program. They are more interested in keeping you "as you were" than in your recovery.
2. Drinking friends have only one friend – their booze. Their drinking habit is more important to them than you are. Let them go.
3. Emotionally healthy individuals are not drawn to relationships with addicted people. If you want an emotionally healthy relationship, begin by becoming emotionally healthy yourself. That takes time, at least twelve months, not two weeks.
4. Your most important friend is your-self. If you can't be *happy* being alone with yourself, no one else can be happy with you either. The key work here is "happy". It's easy to be alone when we are down in the dumps, negative, feeling awful, and have low self esteem. As you begin filling your time with healthy activities and healthy people, your "happiness quotient" will rise.

5. You've just given up your best ally and friend - alcohol. If you stay home, moping and grieving about your loss, you'll soon give in to it and drink again. Get out of the house and get active.

6. If you are single, avoid the trap of new romantic relationships for at least twelve months, or longer, into recovery. Early in your recovery your judgment will be clouded and distorted. You will most likely attract the very problems you are trying to avoid. The relationship you want to build is with yourself, falling in love with new you.

Next, let's think about support.

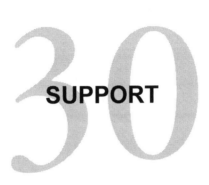

# SUPPORT

Support may be the single most important resource you can have. Any recovery program is bound to be difficult, to say the least, because the changes required for recovery dip deeply into one's emotional life, belief systems, history, and physical memory, as well into deeply ingrained habits and behaviors.

After years of self-denial and rationalization, the mind doesn't want to let go. The mind has been less than truthful with itself and others in order to survive. It's a normal reaction. Don't be too upset about it or even take the time to defend it. It's just the way it is. As your brain and body begin to detoxify and your neurotransmitters begin the process of rebuilding, you will soon see daylight and when you do, you will find relief and be glad.

Perhaps the bigger challenge is to feel emotions again. Emotions that were buried while you were drinking will surface like unexpected tidal waves. You may be afraid to experience them and want the comforting blanket of alcohol again. I assure you, the emotions you will experience are bringing you back to life. You will relearn how to handle them just as you once learned how to walk, fall, get up and walk again. You'll find your balance as long as you give yourself time, patience and most of all, acceptance of yourself just as you are, an imperfectly wonderful human being.

During this time it is IMPORTANT TO HAVE A SUPPORT PERSON. Your recovery DEPENDS ON IT. This is a person who will be available to you 24/7. I mean that most seriously. Find a person you can absolutely trust, a person you are comfortable calling at midnight or four in the morning, if needed. And CALL whenever you begin craving, or if you are thinking of quitting or are having thoughts of suicide. There's really nothing wrong with you.

Remember, it's your neurotransmitter deficiencies and hypoglycemia that are making you feel this way. This is not the real you. CALL YOUR SUPPORT and get help to ride through this shaky period of your recovery. Your support person WANTS you to call. Do it.

Your support person is not your teacher or your therapist, your best friend or your spouse. This person is your SUPPORT. He or she listens, and listens, and listens, and makes you feel accepted, OK, encouraged, lifted up, motivated and LOVED. And, your support person never hesitates to tell you the truth or give you the feedback you really need.

Please choose a support person who understands this program. That person needs to listen to the CD *Reward Deficiency Syndrome* and read this book in order to walk by your side without conflict.

What about your spouse or partner and other family members? It is most certainly OK if someone else shops for food, fixes your meals and makes sure you get your supplements on time in the early days when your brain and emotions are helter-skelter. As you progress, you can move to coordinating these efforts together and eventually become self-responsible.

My husband, David, and I each have defined tasks we have *chosen* to be responsible for. He takes care of things I'm ignorant about, such as fixing cars. I usually take care of food shopping, meals, washing clothes and so on. But, David will fix meals, shop, and wash clothes whenever I have something else I need to do. He is as capable as I and willingly and joyfully does whatever is needed. He frequently offers to do these chores just because he wants to do them. It's healthy to share responsibilities. Having family support is crucial. Allow your family to assist you with your recovery. That is not co-dependency. They are not enabling you as long as you are on the road to recovery.

Your family needs as much support in recovery as you do. They are suffering from the disease of alcoholism in their own way. Your spouse and children, if you have them, need their separate support people or support groups, as well. Your parents and siblings are also involved in this disease and will benefit from education and support.

I know that, in some cases, one doesn't get this kind of family support. All the more reason to have your own support. You may benefit from a support group as well.

This alcohol recovery program is a *Do-It-Yourself* program and that means YOU are in charge of putting your recovery program together. It doesn't mean you do it alone. You are not alone. Your support person is waiting for you to ask.

Nothing you can ever say about your life is new. It's all been heard before. You will find friends who know exactly what you have experienced and know what you are going through right now. You will find the place where you feel you belong. All you have to do is open the door. Your recovery is waiting for you.

*Your support person is waiting for you to ask.*
*ASK*
*Ask, seek, Knock and it shall be opened to you.*

# REWARD DEFICIENCY SUPPORT GROUPS
# OR RDS SUPPORT GROUPS

I have a vision of a new support group based on the knowledge of the cause of addiction and the all-natural treatment model for long-term successful recovery without relapse.

- It is a group without shame, blame or guilt. Members are not anonymous because there is no need to be.
- It is educational and provides all the information a *newbie* needs to understand and treat their addiction.
- Mentors who have *been there* are immediately available to help and inform newcomers.
- It is always open to the latest scientific research and the latest treatment methods that are producing high levels of recovery.
- It is positive, encouraging and supportive as members go through the stages of biochemical restoration.
- It provides a new understanding family, but doesn't foster dependency.
- It understands *Post Acute Withdrawal Syndrome* (PAWS) and assists recovering individuals as their brain chemistry is in the restoration phase. (Chapter 32.)
- It reaches out to inform and support those who haven't learned about the NEW alcoholism story.
- War stories and comparison stories are outlawed.
- Stories that inspire and guide are welcomed.
- No advice is given. Only one's own story of recovery is shared.
- There are no rules that would cause the support group to stagnate.
- Each group finds its own path.
- There is written and digital information available explaining the real cause of addictions and the successful methods of recovery.
- Outside experts in the addiction field are invited speakers.
- Other resources and educational opportunities are made available to restore psycho/social behaviors.
- Informed speakers go into the community to educate teachers and school children.

- Members from the health community find ways to inform those in the addiction field about more advanced treatments.
- Lists of local resources for energy or body work, therapy, and health care practitioners, who understand RDS, are made available to members.
- Lists of local fresh and organic food suppliers.
- Lists of biochemical recovery programs and treatment facilities are made available.
- Social and family gatherings are sponsored.
- People with all addictions are welcomed.
- It remains apolitical and non-religious.

What suggestions do you have? What is your vision? How can we reach out to educate people to seek early intervention without shame, blame and guilt? How do we end the cycle of relapse? Let's inform the world.

# PART FIVE

## *AFTERCARE*

# PAWS AND AD(H)D

JAKE completed 30 days of a residential rehab program following two DUIs. At age 27, he was determined to get his life straightened out. He had a supportive wife who was expecting their first baby. Jake had always had a reading problem, poor comprehension, and difficulty paying attention in classes. Even though he tried to pay attention in group sessions, he was easily distracted.

Still, Jake gave the program his all. On the day of graduation from treatment, he proudly presented his wife with a certificate of completion and a well-won medal. One month later Jake was drinking heavily again. He couldn't handle the stress, his inability to focus and concentrate, and the mood swings.

Jake had Attention Deficit Disorder but it had never been diagnosed. He had learned that alcohol helped him to focus. His performance at work improved with a little alcohol in his system. Mostly, the stress of daily living, making decisions, family expectations, and his concern about taking care of a growing family was just too much.

Was Jake's relapse his fault? No. Failure to identify the underlying cause of his alcoholism, biochemical imbalances – including ADD, was a surefire route to his relapse.

Jake had PAWS (Post Acute Withdrawal Syndrome) which is often the same as symptoms of AD(H)D. The traditional recovery system let him down. PAWS education was not a part of the treatment program, nor was it understood that many alcoholics are self-medicating AD(H)D with alcohol.

Fortunately, Jake found another treatment program that focused on restoring his brain chemical imbalances and addressed the ADD. He learned about PAWS but found that when he stayed with his supplement program, his stress level was much reduced and he could manage the ADD symptoms. Jake is no longer an alcoholic. He enjoys playing with his daughter and is looking forward to the birth of his second baby. Jake's marriage is happy and he is able to perform well at his job.

LYNN, a 44 year old mother of three, was more fortunate. Lynn drank and smoked marijuana before entering a treatment program. She didn't have AD(H)D and her treatment program educated her about PAWS. Lynn stuck to her supplement schedule for fifteen months and rarely had any symptoms of PAWS. Her recovery was smooth and relapse-free.

So, let's take a look at PAWS. The symptoms listed below are common for those who do nothing to repair imbalanced brain chemistry. When you follow a biochemical restoration recovery program, you will reduce or eliminate most or all of these symptoms.

## POST ACUTE WITHDRAWAL SYNDROME

The symptoms of PAWS are psycho-motor reactions that occur intermittently as a result of stimuli within the primitive brain. They usually begin about two weeks after one stops drinking. Alcohol will relieve the symptoms and that's why so many people who stop drinking *without nutrient support* relapse so quickly.

These symptoms can't be consciously controlled. They are coming from the Reward Pathway, as well as from the neurotransmitters that are still unbalanced. Be kind to yourself and continue your nutrient support. The "old" automatic brain is learning to adjust to different stimuli, and it takes times to reorient. Be patient. Don't judge, blame or guilt yourself. This is important. It takes time to rebuild your brain chemistry.

Plan to continue taking the food supplements and remain on the nutritional plan for a year to two years, if necessary, in order to avoid the majority of PAWS symptoms.

**The nutrient support you are receiving in this program decreases or eliminates most of these symptoms.**

## DEFINITION

PAWS is a set of symptoms that begin after detoxifying from alcohol. It lasts for 12 to 24 months. PAWS is caused by withdrawal from the alcohol, and it doesn't seem to be affected by the length of time one was drinking.

## PHYSICAL PROBLEMS

1. All the senses are easily over-stimulated. Smells, taste, touch, hearing and vision are affected. A smell can bring back a memory, taste can stimulate craving, noise may irritate you, you may over-react to touch, and sights may stimulate memories and emotions. People can over-react to any of these sensual stimuli.
2. Depression can be caused by changes in the brain chemistry. If you continue with your supplements and nutritional guidelines this should not be the problem for you. Problems occur when people stop their recovery program prematurely or don't follow the program as directed. Type A people like to design their own course of action, but this program does not allow for independent creativity. Work the program as designed for success.
3. Without the supplements, people experience increased stress. As your brain chemistry is being restored, you will be able to handle stress better. Remember to take your GABA.

## MENTAL PROBLEMS

1. There may be poor concentration and difficulty with listening. Take L-Tyrosine.
2. Untreated brain chemistry creates rigid, repetitive thinking and it's difficult to turn thoughts off. Try adding Inositol, a B vitamin.
3. The ability of abstract thinking is impaired.
4. It's difficult to sort out "cause and effect".

## MEMORY PROBLEMS

1. Memories don't move from short to long term.
2. Memories cause increased stress.

## EMOTIONAL PROBLEMS

1. There are overreactions and under-reactions to life circumstances. GABA helps.
2. Emotional reactions occur without apparent stimulus. Use DLPA.
3. Mood swings occur at any time without reason. 5HTP for Serotonin.
4. Increased stress is felt more frequently (again).
5. Sudden panic can occur. Take the vitamin Inositol.

## SLEEP DISTURBANCE PROBLEMS

1. There may be frequent nightmares.
2. Increased dreaming can occur.
3. There may be difficulty falling or staying asleep. 5 HTP plus GABA
4. Sometimes there is a feeling of always being tired.
5. Increased stress is felt (again).

## PSYCHOMOTOR PROBLEMS

1. You may feel dizzy, clumsy, or unsteady. Take L-Glutamine.
2. Reflexes may be slow and there may be poor hand/eye coordination.
3. Increased stress (again).

## STRESS

1. There can be difficulty determining high from low emotional stress.
   Stress causes all other symptoms to worsen. Take GABA, L-Glutamine and Inositol.
2. Stress causes increased PAWS –
   which causes increased STRESS –
   which causes increased PAWS –
   which causes increased STRESS!!!

## ATTENTION DEFICIT DISORDER (ADD)
## ATTENTION DEFICIT HYPERACTIVITY DISORDER (ADHD)

It is estimated by some that as many as 50% to 70% of alcoholics have *undiagnosed* AD(H)D.[1] This estimate makes sense because the PAWS symptoms are so common among recovering alcoholics. You see, PAWS and AD(H)D symptoms are almost identical. Let's compare.

## ATTENTION DEFICIT DISORDER

Common symptoms:

- Poor listener
- Losing things
- Easily distracted
- Poor organization
- Lack of sustained attention
- Forgetful in daily activities
- Failure to follow through on tasks
- Careless mistakes/lack of attention to details
- Avoiding tasks requiring sustained mental effort

## ATTENTION DEFICIT HYPERACTIVE DISORDER

Common symptoms includes all of the above plus:

- Intrusive
- "On the go"
- Leaving seat
- Can't wait turn
- Excessive talking
- Fidgeting/squirming
- Blurting out answers
- Excessive running/climbing
- Difficulty with quiet activities

If teenagers have primary RDS and are experiencing some of these symptoms, alcohol provides a welcome and rewarding relief that will eventually lead to an addiction. When they stop drinking, perhaps years later, all the undiagnosed symptoms quickly return, usually within two weeks of abstinence. AD(H)D can never be completely cured. Adults with AD(H)D learn how to adapt and cope but continue to suffer from symptoms.

If a person with AD(H)D was undiagnosed before the drinking began, then the reoccurrence of the symptoms can be so disconcerting and prevalent that alcohol will be a welcome relief, no matter how motivated the person is to recover. (Symptoms are greatly alleviated when imbalanced brain chemistry is restored.)

### *If recovery means feeling worse, then who needs it?*

It's amazing that traditional treatment programs are not addressing PAWS for what it is. The good news is that if you have PAWS after completing your program, it will be to a much lesser degree and much more manageable than if you had quit drinking "cold turkey".

The rebalancing of your neurotransmitter chemistry goes a long way to reducing the symptoms of both PAWS and AD(H)D.

If you don't have AD(H)D you will move through your recovery with little or no symptoms *provided* you followed the supplement and nutrition program carefully.

If you *do* have ADD/ ADHD, your symptoms, while always there, will be greatly reduced. I highly recommend the book *Overload: Attention Deficit Disorder and the Addictive Brain* by David Miller and Kenneth Blum, PhD, (the same neuroscientist who discovered and named RDS). In this book, Blum explains RDS and the story behind the discovery of the genetic code for neurotransmitter deficiencies.

David Miller has AD(H)D and gives a compassionate and accurate portrait of what's it like to have this disorder, as well as suggestions for making one's life easier.

HINT: L-Tyrosine will be your best friend, accompanied by the relaxing GABA, L-Taurine, and L-Theonine.

## SOLUTION TO PAWS:
## PSYCHO-SPIRITUAL HEALTH MAINTENANCE

1. Find a personal mentor, a person you look up to and admire. Make sure this person understands what the real cause of addiction is and will eagerly support you in your biochemical restoration program, as well as with all the other pieces of your recovery.

2. Pay strong attention to your spiritual program, whatever that might be. Alcoholics usually lose sight of their inner connection with Source. Follow your intuition and listen to your heart. Don't let old religious ideas about addiction control you. Remember, this is the NEW alcoholism story, and you are on the cutting edge of what is working.

3. Nurture family relations. They have usually suffered as a result of the addiction. Others were negatively affected by your behaviors. It is important to forgive yourself and ask for their understanding and forgiveness. Making amends in any manner that is healthy and acceptable to others will help you to forgive yourself. Hopefully, your family has participated in your recovery program and is ready to move forward. What if your family doesn't get it? Move forward. Use your resources of support person, support group, and the new friends you are developing as you go to your new activities.

4. Educate and help others to recover. This may be the best guidance that you can have for your recovery.

5. Meditate and follow your Bliss.

## PHYSICAL HEALTH MAINTENANCE

By following this program, PAWS may never be much of a challenge for you. Stray off the program and you will most likely be back in the PAWS of alcohol.

1. Continue the nutrient formulas for one to two years.
2. Maintain your healthy nutritional program.
3. Get a sauna occasionally.
4. Maintain regular exercise
5. Continue receiving frequent massages. This is a very important step to keep the stress level under control as well as removing the toxins that continue to assault all of us.
6. Drink eight glasses of water daily.
7. Get six to eight hours of sleep nightly.
8. Stop smoking or chewing tobacco.

YOU CAN DO IT

Is all this doable? Well...,

Is alcohol addiction doable?

Which is more difficult?

What do you want?

First, let's agree, (now that you know about the real cause of addictions,) that you have nothing to be ashamed about. You didn't ask for or cause this disease to happen. It won't go away by itself. It will progress if not addressed.

That said, if all this information has given you a *"go"* message, then order your supplements and begin your recovery program. You can do it. You can have the life you were born to have, free of addiction and all the negative side effects. Relapse no more.

## AAA
## AMINO ACID ADDICT
## AMINOS ARE THE ANTIDOTE

# 33
# RELAPSE NO MORE

## CHANGE YOUR THINKING

*"I'm not an alcoholic."*
*"I used to be an alcoholic."*
*"I will become an alcoholic if I drink again."*
*"I'm not just sober. I'm recovered."*

"My name is Matt and I'm an alcoholic. Alcoholics drink. Alcoholics struggle, one day at a time, to stay sober. 'Easy does it' 'cause it's easy to drink again. Alcoholics relapse. Sober alcoholics experience cravings, depression, irritability, insomnia, anxiety, and angry outbursts. Sober alcoholics are addicted to caffeine and nicotine, sugar and sodas, and anything sweet. Alcoholics need meetings to stay sober."

When you call yourself an "alcoholic" you're into "stinkin' thinkin' ". You immediately acquire heavy baggage that will weigh you down. If you are not drinking and you are in the process of recovering, shift your thinking to "I'm a healthy and happy person."   Never call yourself an "alcoholic" again as long as you are not drinking.

When you think of being healthy and happy, what goes through your mind?  Instead of struggling to avoid relapse, there's an easyness to life, a flow of goodness and joy.

Isn't this what you want?  So, fill your mind with thoughts of the good life you intend to have, you expect to have, and you are creating right now. Once you have stopped drinking AND are in the process of restoring your brain chemistry, you are NOT an alcoholic any more.

*"I was an alcoholic and I've recovered. I'm not an alcoholic anymore."*

## IMAGINE

Imagine the life you want. Imagination is the first step to creating the rest of your life. All things are possible – no limits – except those you impose upon yourself. Of course, we have to be realistic. I'm not going to be an astronaut, much as I might want to. But I jumped out of an airplane at 18,000 feet and felt the exhilaration of being free in space.

Who do you want to be? What do you want to achieve? Where do you want to go? Who do you want to share your life with? Imagine it all without any reservations or judgments.

Which of those imaginations makes your heart leap? What is your wildest dream? Dare to dream and dare to believe that you are capable of achieving anything you put your heart and soul into.

## VISUALIZE

See your imaginings taking shape within your mind. See where they take you. See the colors and textures, the shades and hues. Let your mind see into the future, a future you are creating by choice, not accident.

There are no accidents. We create our future just as we have created our past. What we fear, comes to us. What we desire with intention and expectation, comes to us. Put your energy in what you want, not what you don't want. Put a new vision of life into your mind, one with only good in it.

## FEEL

What does your chosen future feel like in your body? Does your heart sing? Does it bring a smile to your face? Can you feel laughter and happiness in your chest? Soak up and wallow in good feelings. Feel NOW what your chosen future holds for you.

Smile and be grateful for all the good that is coming into your life, RIGHT NOW. You may not see it in the physical yet, but I assure you, as you imagine, visualize, and feel it to be true, so it is.

Be patient. Your chosen future will manifest in the right time under the right circumstances. Hold on to your dream. Let no one meddle with your dream. Tell only those who will share the dream with the same belief that you have.

## BREATHE IT

Imagine, visualize, and feel your chosen future as you breathe it all deeply into your solar-plexus. Let your rib cage expand as it fills with the joy and freedom and good health and clear thinking and taste of life you are breathing in right now. Continue to breathe in and experience and live the life you are choosing and the life you are expecting and the life you know is coming to you.

## PROTECTIVE BUBBLE

Visualize a Plexiglas bubble around you that protects you from all negativity, and all temptations that might move you out of your inner knowing. Love flows through this bubble but no negativity can pass through it to you. Any negativity that hits the bubble simply bounces back to the sender, where it belongs.

No one knows the bubble is there except you. Put it around you every morning and go about your business. You will discover that this bubble is real and it works.

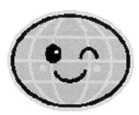

ALCOHOLIC NO MORE

# RECOVERY PROGRAM SUMMARY

Make your recovery program a way of life for twelve to twenty-four months. These first weeks are only the beginning. It takes many months for your brain chemistry to normalize. Indeed, it may never completely normalize. Taking your micronutrients and continuing to eat three nutritious meals daily has to become a way of life, for life.

Over time, you will adjust your micronutrients as needed, but continue taking them on schedule for twelve to twenty-four months. After your brain chemistry and life are stabilized, create a maintenance program for a relapse-free life.

"STINKIN' THINKIN' " IS WHEN YOU BEGIN TO FEEL GREAT AND
THINK YOU CAN QUIT TAKING YOUR SUPPLEMENTS.
IF YOU DO QUIT – HELLO RELAPSE!
(See NOTE at end of chapter.)

## SEVEN STEPS TO RECOVERY

1. Amino Acids
2. Food Supplements
3. Nutrition
4. Saunas
5. Massage
6. Exercise
7. Support

## CHECKLISTS

In the next section you will find Weekly checklists to help you stay on track and monitor your progress.

## JOURNALING

Keep a daily journal. This is a huge help as the days go by. After a time you won't remember how you felt in the past. Rereading your journal will show you just how much improvement you are making.

Your journal doesn't have to be a diary. Just jot down how you are feeling physically, emotionally, and spiritually. Make a note of any new ideas, awarenesses, and "aha" moments.

You are about to take a big step to recovery. I assure you that by using a biochemical approach, you will have the best opportunity for long-lasting recovery you can possibly have. Whether you decide to use this *Do-It-Yourself Program* or go to a treatment facility that follows the same approach, you are going to receive the best and most advanced scientific care available.

## WHAT'S THE CATCH?

TOM, a recent college graduate, was hired by a well known engineering firm and he had a good future in front of him. He liked his new job and was getting good feedback about his work. Tom followed his recovery program almost perfectly for two months. He felt the best he had felt in years and he had no cravings. In fact, he felt so good that he quit taking his supplements because he didn't think he needed them anymore. Two weeks later he was drinking again, even more than before. Tom has become an alcoholic again and his new job is in jeopardy.

MARIE is married and works two jobs so that she and her husband can continue to send their two boys to college. She is so stressed and tired that she doesn't eat as well as she would like and many times misses her recovery nutrients. Yet, she continues to follow her recovery program as best she can. She is determined not to give up. Now into her second month on the program, she is sleeping a little better and she's noticing that her anxiety is less. Her husband has noticed that she laughs more and doesn't seem quite as worried as she used be. Marie says she isn't missing her alcohol any more. Even though Marie got off to a slow and spotty start, she is feeling better, handling the stress better, and has decided to follow the recovery program more closely.

SEAN stuck to his recovery program even though his wife decided to leave him shortly after he started the program. She didn't believe a nutritional method of recovery would work. After four weeks on the program Sean felt well enough to seek counseling. Two months later his wife decided to go into counseling, as well. Seven months later, Sean's wife felt he was serious about his recovery and that maybe the program was working after all, so she moved back home with him. Now, they are working together to create a better relationship and both feel hopeful that things are going to work out. If all continues to go well, they are talking about creating a family in the future, but they want to focus on their recovery and relationship first.

RACHAEL had a low paying job and a seven year old son to care for. Still, she did the best she could. She bought the aminos and the vitamin supplements. She couldn't afford the massages and didn't have the money to join a YMCA. However, she set about walking every day, no matter what the weather was. She cut out her usual coffee and doughnut in the morning and started to eat more protein and fat with most every meal. As she started to eat better, and feed her son better, Rachael noticed his behaviors improved, as well. She was afraid to stop the program because she didn't want her son to have a drunkard for a mother. Ten months later Rachael is still following the program. She says sticking to the recovery program has just become a natural part of her life. She is functioning so much better at work that she was given a better job and a raise in pay. She celebrated by taking her son on a weekend camping trip where they had a great time. Rachael is on her way to a healthy recovery.

## YOUR RECOVERY PROGRAM

This *early intervention* Do-It-Yourself Recovery Program is a TWELVE to TWENTY FOUR month program. That means continuing to take your supplements and aminos while maintaining your healthy nutritional program for twelve to twenty-four months.

Studies show that individuals who attend a 28 day residential treatment program, of any kind, have an almost immediate relapse rate. Most residential treatment programs are now 60 and 90 day programs with follow-up support. Even then, the relapse rates are up to 95% because 1) the programs don't change the underlying brain chemistry, and 2), client's don't stick with the program elements after leaving the residential program.

Just think, while in the program, all medications are provided by a nurse at specific times and the clients are expected to be present to get those medications. Clients never have to shop for food or prepare their meals. In this program you are the one in charge of taking your micronutrients and eating three healthy meals a day. No one is there to make you be compliant.

This is why you must be highly motivated and functional in order to do this program, not for just a couple of months, but for the "long haul". However, this "long haul" is being done in a "Rolls Royce" program, one that can remove the underlying cause of your addiction when followed.

## QUESTIONS

These are some of the questions I get when people call me about doing this program. They are valid questions so I want to answer them in this book because they might be questions that you have, as well.

*"I've been drinking every day for almost forty years. Will this program help me?"*

I'll tell you about two of my clients who have been drinking for forty or more years. (I've changed the names and some of the details to protect their privacy.)

I'll call the first client Deborah. She was an 80 year old, energetic and active woman who drank at least four or five glasses of wine every evening. Deborah had an organic garden, grew her own vegetables and ate in a very healthy manner. She had never stopped drinking or tried to quit before calling me. However, she wanted to make sure she remained healthy for the rest of her life and so Deborah decided to quit drinking. Her only medication was for high blood pressure. Deborah took to the Do-It-Yourself Managed Recovery Program with ease. She had no withdrawal symptoms, and soon felt great. Even though some of her friends continued to drink while visiting her, she never drank again and had no cravings. I suspect that Deborah had been *abusing* alcohol versus being addicted to it. The ease of her recovery suggests that she didn't have a *reward deficiency* or she had only a *slight deficiency* which was quickly normalized with the amino acids and micronutrient protocol. Her blood pressure remained high, however, and she had to continue taking her blood pressure medication.

I'll call the second client, Stan. At age 56, Stan had been drinking since age sixteen. He drank heavily and had been to two treatment programs, one of which was an Intensive Outpatient Program. Stan had attended AA for two years and gave it up in frustration over not being able to quit drinking. Stan owns and still runs his own auto repair business. When his wife reached the point of total frustration, worry, and fear of losing him, he "agreed" to try the Do-It-Yourself Managed Program. (Agreeing to do a recovery program for someone else is a sure-fire program for relapse.) Stan has high blood pressure and high blood sugar levels but refuses to take any medication. He followed the program faithfully for five weeks and began to "feel great", in his own words. He rarely thought about drinking. His energy level was up and he was sleeping better. Then his wife went to visit their daughter in another state for a few days. Bingo! Stan didn't follow his amino and supplement schedule for a couple of days. Then he bought a bottle of whisky and drank it. He was remorseful and determined never to do that again. Back on the recovery program, wanting to quit, but still drinking "a few drops" every two or three days, he continues to follow the program and hopes it will work. I encouraged him to take the medicine his physician prescribed for his blood pressure and elevated blood sugar but Stan refuses. Given the triggers that send Stan to the liquor store, and his non-compliance with the medication, I recommended that Stan go into a 90 day residential treatment program. He says he realizes that he may have to do that some day, but not now. Now Stan is more than ever motivated to quit drinking and follows the recovery program closely, but his primitive brain is so responsive to *drinking triggers* that the Do-It-Yourself Recovery Program may not work for him. On the other hand, maybe he will rebuild his brain chemistry enough over time that recovery will become easier for him and he will eventually fully recover on this program. I hope so. Time will tell.

### *"I've been through three residential treatment programs and relapsed every time. Will this program work for me?"*

Like Stan, someone who has relapsed multiple times over several years has so many *drinking triggers* that a do-it-yourself recovery program will most likely not work. This program is an early intervention program for highly motivated, highly functioning individuals. Someone like Deborah, who probably was abusing but not addicted to alcohol can benefit from this program but for a long-term addiction, I recommend a 90 day residential program that specializes in biochemical recovery. Obviously, the treatment programs that didn't address Stan's underlying biochemical imbalances didn't work for him.

### *"I'm on a limited budget. How can I do this program?"*

Jason was introduced to this program by someone who had read my first book, *The NEW Alcoholism Story Everyone Needs to Know*. She called me and asked for assistance in helping Jason. Jason was not able to purchase all the supplements and amino acids but he bought what he could afford and followed the program with enthusiasm, not drinking, and feeling great. He was very pleased and proud of his accomplishment. However, after three months, even with his friend's support, he started drinking again. Without all of the micronutrients, Jason's brain chemistry was unable to restore itself. That said, everyone is different. We don't know why Jason relapsed. Another person may have continued on and recovered fully, even without being able to take all the supplements. What are the stressors? Jason had severe relationship issues and his personal life was filled with drama. What was his level of *reward deficiency*? A low deficiency level is more easily resolved than a high deficiency level. Did he have all the support he needed? Did Jason have medical or mental health issues aside from the addiction? Because he didn't work directly with me, I don't have his background information. For those who have a limited budget and can't afford a residential or outpatient program, or can't find one that repairs brain chemistry, do the best you can on this program. Whatever you do will be better than going "cold turkey". Even doing a little bit of this program may be all you need to recover. The most important recommendation I can give to start and stick with whatever you can afford. You can always call for a consultation to create a program that fits your budget. Once you start, don't give up.

### *"I work nights and sleep during the day. How can I do this program?"*

Working nights is very hard on the brain and body but some of us have to do it. Years ago I worked night-shifts as a nurse and know the toll it takes. The good news is that you can still work this program. Make sure you eat three meals well-spaced as if it were daytime. Take your supplements before, with, and between meals as directed. Just move the schedule up to the time when you get up during the day. The more difficult time is on your "off" days. Whenever you wake up, start the schedule with the "before breakfast" aminos and carry on from there.

### *"Can I work this program even if my wife (or husband) doesn't want to quit drinking?"*

You can certainly begin the program but the odds are stacked against success. I suggest that you do some serious thinking about your relationship and the future you want. Trying to remain sober with a drinking partner is about impossible. Even attempting to recover together is difficult. That's why husband and wife are separated in treatment programs. I suggest some counseling with a qualified family therapist to sort out your thinking.

### "My seventeen year old son needs help. Will this program work for him?"

That's a huge question. To begin, teenagers are oppositional and non-compliant by nature. Their socialization stops at the age when they begin serious drinking. Their brains aren't fully developed until about age 26 even without drinking. I frequently get calls from terrified parents. But why isn't the "son" or "daughter" calling me? We can't fix our children, as much as we would like to. Teenagers may say they want to quit drinking (rarely) but they really don't want to quit. Even though they may have been exposed to the results of drinking in the family, the teen thinks he or she is different. Until the repercussions of drinking hit home where it hurts, they usually won't be willing to give up their "exciting" life. It would be a rare teen who can be compliant with this program. At this young age, the best treatment would be a *long* residential program that provides a biochemical approach. For the names and locations of these programs, contact me through www.BrainworksAlcoholRecovery.com. Meanwhile, make sure there is no alcohol in your home and take away the teen's driving privileges. Know where your teen is and keep him or her busy. Seek counseling for yourself, as a parent.

### "Can I do this program if I'm on a medication for anxiety, (or depression), and drinking too?"

Research studies are showing that all medications for mood and mental disorders including antidepressants, benzodiazepines, and antipsychotics, are highly addictive and increase the likelihood of making the original condition *chronic over time*, similar to the results of long term drinking. Drinking while taking any of these medications can have serious side effects including overdosing and/or suicide. This program can be followed in conjunction with careful withdrawal from these medications under your healthcare provider's direction. Take this manual to your physician and request assistance. Be aware that the majority of physicians are totally ignorant about nutrition, brain biochemistry, and addiction. Find a healthcare provider that understands this program and who will work with you to achieve your recovery. Be assertive, ask for what YOU want, and keep going until you find the healthcare provider that can work well with you.

### "I'm a diabetic and have high blood pressure. Is it safe to do this program?"

This program will improve your overall health. Alcohol use elevates blood pressure and promotes diabetes. The nutritional plan in this program helps to normalize both blood sugar and blood pressure. Continue to follow your healthcare provider's advice, monitor your blood pressure and blood sugar frequently, and make adjustments in the medication you are taking as necessary. Many people are able to reduce or give up these medications within a very short time after starting this program.

### "I'm calling about my husband, (son), (daughter), (mother)... Can this program help him?"

I find that the people who benefit the most from this program are the ones who are seeking a solution themselves. They are highly motivated. They are searching the web, going to the library or bookstore, or are asking the questions. If you think this program is right for a family member or friends, tell them about it and let them call for information. If they don't have enough interest to call, they aren't ready, aren't motivated, or this program doesn't resonate with their belief system. When someone calls me about another person I'm happy to answer their questions and I always end the conversation by saying that the next step is for the person in question to call me him or herself.

Do you have questions that I haven't answered in this book? If so, just call me and ask. I want to help you, or your loved one, to recover.

## OVERWHELMED BY ALL THIS?

If you are feeling a bit overwhelmed by everything you've read in this book, it's OK. Don't give up. Go to www.BrainworksAlcoholRecovery.com and request either a consultation or a Managed Program (See Appendix A). I'll be happy to answer your questions and guide you through the program. Coaching by telephone with my husband, David Horst, is also available for motivation, help with life-style issues, and support.

That's it. Your recovery is very important to us, as well as to you and your loved ones. You will be doing the program in your home but you will not be alone. We hold you in our hearts.

NOTE: *What should I do if I do relapse?*
Good question, but you already know what to do. Stop fretting and making excuses. No shame, no blame, no guilt. Your triggers got to you, or you stopped following your recovery program, or you thought you were already recovered. Take stock, learn from this experience, and get right back on your recovery program. Call Dr. Suka for guidance and support if you like.

# CHECK LISTS AND WORK SHEETS

SYMPTOM CHECKLIST WEEK THREE                          Date_____

INSTRUCTIONS:  Put a number from **zero** (no symptoms) to **ten** for each symptom you have, with **one being slightly felt or hardly ever felt** and **ten being strongly felt or felt all the time.**

_____ Cravings for alcohol

_____ Uses alcohol regularly

_____ Tendency to allergies, asthma, hay fever, rashes

_____ Bad dreams

_____ No dream recall

_____ Unstable moods, frequent mood swings

_____ Blurred vision

_____ Frequent thirst

_____ Bruises easily

_____ Confusion

_____ Nervous stomach

_____ Poor sleep, insomnia, waking up during the night

_____ Nervous exhaustion

_____ Indecision

_____ Can't work under pressure

_____ Cravings for sweets

_____ Depression

_____ Feelings of suspicion, paranoia

_____ Light-headedness, dizziness

_____ Anxiety

_____ Fearfulness

## SYMPTOM CHECKLIST WEEK THREE continued

_____ Tremors, shakes

_____ Night sweats

_____ Heart palpitations

_____ Compulsive, obsessive, driven

_____ Manic-depressive (cyclical mood changes)

_____ Suicidal thoughts

_____ Irritability, sudden anger

_____ Lack of energy

_____ Magnifies insignificant events

_____ Poor memory

_____ Inability to concentrate

_____ Sleepy after meals or late in the afternoon

_____ Chronic worrier

_____ Difficulty awakening in the morning

TOTAL THE NUMBERS FOR YOUR SCORE: _____

Adapted from *Seven Weeks to Sobriety* by Joan Mathews Larson, PhD

SYMPTOM CHECKLIST WEEK SIX                    Date_____

INSTRUCTIONS:  Put a number from **zero** (no symptoms) to **ten** for each symptom you have, with **one being slightly felt or hardly ever felt** and **ten being strongly felt or felt all the time.**

_____ Cravings for alcohol

_____ Uses alcohol regularly

_____ Tendency to allergies, asthma, hay fever, rashes

_____ Bad dreams

_____ No dream recall

_____ Unstable moods, frequent mood swings

_____ Blurred vision

_____ Frequent thirst

_____ Bruises easily

_____ Confusion

_____ Nervous stomach

_____ Poor sleep, insomnia, waking up during the night

_____ Nervous exhaustion

_____ Indecision

_____ Can't work under pressure

_____ Cravings for sweets

_____ Depression

_____ Feelings of suspicion, paranoia

_____ Light-headedness, dizziness

_____ Anxiety

_____ Fearfulness

## SYMPTOM CHECKLIST WEEK SIX  continued

_____ Tremors, shakes

_____ Night sweats

_____ Heart palpitations

_____ Compulsive, obsessive, driven

_____ Manic-depressive (cyclical mood changes)

_____ Suicidal thoughts

_____ Irritability, sudden anger

_____ Lack of energy

_____ Magnifies insignificant events

_____ Poor memory

_____ Inability to concentrate

_____ Sleepy after meals or late in the afternoon

_____ Chronic worrier

_____ Difficulty awakening in the morning


TOTAL THE NUMBERS FOR YOUR SCORE: _____


Adapted from *Seven Weeks to Sobriety* by Joan Mathews Larson, PhD

SYMPTOM CHECKLIST THREE MONTHS                    Date_____

INSTRUCTIONS:  Put a number from **zero** (no symptoms) to **ten** for each symptom you have, with **one being slightly felt or hardly ever felt** and **ten being strongly felt or felt all the time.**

_____ Cravings for alcohol

_____ Uses alcohol regularly

_____ Tendency to allergies, asthma, hay fever, rashes

_____ Bad dreams

_____ No dream recall

_____ Unstable moods, frequent mood swings

_____ Blurred vision

_____ Frequent thirst

_____ Bruises easily

_____ Confusion

_____ Nervous stomach

_____ Poor sleep, insomnia, waking up during the night

_____ Nervous exhaustion

_____ Indecision

_____ Can't work under pressure

_____ Cravings for sweets

_____ Depression

_____ Feelings of suspicion, paranoia

_____ Light-headedness, dizziness

_____ Anxiety

_____ Fearfulness

## SYMPTOM CHECKLIST THREE MONTHS  continued

_____ Tremors, shakes

_____ Night sweats

_____ Heart palpitations

_____ Compulsive, obsessive, driven

_____ Manic-depressive (cyclical mood changes)

_____ Suicidal thoughts

_____ Irritability, sudden anger

_____ Lack of energy

_____ Magnifies insignificant events

_____ Poor memory

_____ Inability to concentrate

_____ Sleepy after meals or late in the afternoon

_____ Chronic worrier

_____ Difficulty awakening in the morning


TOTAL THE NUMBERS FOR YOUR SCORE: _____


Adapted from *Seven Weeks to Sobriety* by Joan Mathews Larson, PhD

SYMPTOM CHECKLIST SIX MONTHS                     Date_____

INSTRUCTIONS: Put a number from **zero** (no symptoms) to **ten** for each symptom you have, with **one being slightly felt or hardly ever felt** and **ten being strongly felt or felt all the time.**

_____ Cravings for alcohol

_____ Uses alcohol regularly

_____ Tendency to allergies, asthma, hay fever, rashes

_____ Bad dreams

_____ No dream recall

_____ Unstable moods, frequent mood swings

_____ Blurred vision

_____ Frequent thirst

_____ Bruises easily

_____ Confusion

_____ Nervous stomach

_____ Poor sleep, insomnia, waking up during the night

_____ Nervous exhaustion

_____ Indecision

_____ Can't work under pressure

_____ Cravings for sweets

_____ Depression

_____ Feelings of suspicion, paranoia

_____ Light-headedness, dizziness

_____ Anxiety

_____ Fearfulness

# SYMPTOM CHECKLIST SIX MONTHS continued

_____ Tremors, shakes

_____ Night sweats

_____ Heart palpitations

_____ Compulsive, obsessive, driven

_____ Manic-depressive (cyclical mood changes)

_____ Suicidal thoughts

_____ Irritability, sudden anger

_____ Lack of energy

_____ Magnifies insignificant events

_____ Poor memory

_____ Inability to concentrate

_____ Sleepy after meals or late in the afternoon

_____ Chronic worrier

_____ Difficulty awakening in the morning

TOTAL THE NUMBERS FOR YOUR SCORE: _____

Adapted from *Seven Weeks to Sobriety* by Joan Mathews Larson, PhD

# WEEKLY SCHEDULE

Using the daily checklists on the following pages for nine weeks will help to set the pattern for the rest of your recovery months. Just number the weeks and add in the dates. Place a checkmark for each activity you completed under the day that you completed it.

These checklists will keep you on track. As you look at these checklists over time, you will feel pride in your commitment and dedication to your recovery.

WEEKLY SCHEDULE       WEEK # _____       DATES _____

| ACTIVITIES | Mon | Tue | Wed | Thu | Fri | Sat | Sun |
|---|---|---|---|---|---|---|---|
| 3 Daily Meals | —— | —— | —— | —— | —— | —— | —— |
| 3 Daily Snacks | —— | —— | —— | —— | —— | —— | —— |
| Nutrients as Scheduled | —— | —— | —— | —— | —— | —— | —— |
| 40 Minutes Exercise (4 Times Weekly) | —— | —— | —— | —— | —— | —— | —— |
| Sauna | —— | —— | —— | —— | —— | —— | —— |
| Yoga, Tai Chi, Qigong | —— | —— | —— | —— | —— | —— | —— |
| Homework: Reading, Journaling, etc. | —— | —— | —— | —— | —— | —— | —— |
| Food Planning, Shopping | —— | —— | —— | —— | —— | —— | —— |
| Meal Preparation | —— | —— | —— | —— | —— | —— | —— |
| Quality Family Relations | —— | —— | —— | —— | —— | —— | —— |
| Quality Support Time | —— | —— | —— | —— | —— | —— | —— |
| Fun, Relaxation | —— | —— | —— | —— | —— | —— | —— |

WEEKLY SCHEDULE          WEEK # _____          DATES _____

| ACTIVITIES | Mon | Tue | Wed | Thu | Fri | Sat | Sun |
|---|---|---|---|---|---|---|---|
| 3 Meals Daily | ___ | ___ | ___ | ___ | ___ | ___ | ___ |
| 3 Snacks Daily | ___ | ___ | ___ | ___ | ___ | ___ | ___ |
| Nutrients as Scheduled | ___ | ___ | ___ | ___ | ___ | ___ | ___ |
| 40 Minutes Exercise (4 Times Weekly) | ___ | ___ | ___ | ___ | ___ | ___ | ___ |
| Sauna | ___ | ___ | ___ | ___ | ___ | ___ | ___ |
| Yoga, Tai Chi, Qigong | ___ | ___ | ___ | ___ | ___ | ___ | ___ |
| Homework: Reading, Journaling, etc. | ___ | ___ | ___ | ___ | ___ | ___ | ___ |
| Food Planning, Shopping | ___ | ___ | ___ | ___ | ___ | ___ | ___ |
| Meal Preparation | ___ | ___ | ___ | ___ | ___ | ___ | ___ |
| Quality Family Relations | ___ | ___ | ___ | ___ | ___ | ___ | ___ |
| Quality Support Time | ___ | ___ | ___ | ___ | ___ | ___ | ___ |
| Fun, Relaxation | ___ | ___ | ___ | ___ | ___ | ___ | ___ |
| | ___ | ___ | ___ | ___ | ___ | ___ | ___ |

WEEKLY SCHEDULE          WEEK # _____          DATES _____

| ACTIVITIES | Mon | Tue | Wed | Thu | Fri | Sat | Sun |
|---|---|---|---|---|---|---|---|
| 3 Daily Meals | ____ | ____ | ____ | ____ | ____ | ____ | ____ |
| 3 Daily Snacks | ____ | ____ | ____ | ____ | ____ | ____ | ____ |
| Nutrients as Scheduled | ____ | ____ | ____ | ____ | ____ | ____ | ____ |
| 40 Minutes Exercise (4 Times Weekly) | ____ | ____ | ____ | ____ | ____ | ____ | ____ |
| Sauna | ____ | ____ | ____ | ____ | ____ | ____ | ____ |
| Yoga, Tai Chi, Qigong | ____ | ____ | ____ | ____ | ____ | ____ | ____ |
| Homework: Reading, Journaling, etc. | ____ | ____ | ____ | ____ | ____ | ____ | ____ |
| Food Planning, Shopping | ____ | ____ | ____ | ____ | ____ | ____ | ____ |
| Meal Preparation | ____ | ____ | ____ | ____ | ____ | ____ | ____ |
| Quality Family Relations | ____ | ____ | ____ | ____ | ____ | ____ | ____ |
| Quality Support Time | ____ | ____ | ____ | ____ | ____ | ____ | ____ |
| Quality Alone Time | ____ | ____ | ____ | ____ | ____ | ____ | ____ |
| Fun, Relaxation | ____ | ____ | ____ | ____ | ____ | ____ | ____ |

WEEKLY SCHEDULE          WEEK # _____          DATES _____

| ACTIVITIES | Mon | Tue | Wed | Thu | Fri | Sat | Sun |
|---|---|---|---|---|---|---|---|
| 3 Daily Meals | — | — | — | — | — | — | — |
| 3 Daily Snacks | — | — | — | — | — | — | — |
| Nutrients as Scheduled | — | — | — | — | — | — | — |
| 40 Minutes Exercise (4 Times Weekly) | — | — | — | — | — | — | — |
| Sauna | — | — | — | — | — | — | — |
| Yoga, Tai Chi, Qigong | — | — | — | — | — | — | — |
| Homework: Reading, Journaling, etc. | — | — | — | — | — | — | — |
| Food Planning, Shopping | — | — | — | — | — | — | — |
| Meal Preparation | — | — | — | — | — | — | — |
| Quality Family Relations | — | — | — | — | — | — | — |
| Quality Support Time | — | — | — | — | — | — | — |
| Quality Alone Time | — | — | — | — | — | — | — |
| Fun, Relaxation | — | — | — | — | — | — | — |

WEEKLY SCHEDULE        WEEK # _____        DATES _____

| ACTIVITIES | Mon | Tue | Wed | Thu | Fri | Sat | Sun |
|---|---|---|---|---|---|---|---|
| 3 Daily Meals | — | — | — | — | — | — | — |
| 3 Daily Snacks | — | — | — | — | — | — | — |
| Nutrients as Scheduled | — | — | — | — | — | — | — |
| 40 Minutes Exercise (4 Times Weekly) | — | — | — | — | — | — | — |
| Sauna | — | — | — | — | — | — | — |
| Yoga, Tai Chi, Qigong | — | — | — | — | — | — | — |
| Homework: Reading, Journaling, etc. | — | — | — | — | — | — | — |
| Food Planning, Shopping | — | — | — | — | — | — | — |
| Meal Preparation | — | — | — | — | — | — | — |
| Quality Family Relations | — | — | — | — | — | — | — |
| Quality Support Time | — | — | — | — | — | — | — |
| Quality Alone Time | — | — | — | — | — | — | — |
| Fun, Relaxation | — | — | — | — | — | — | — |

WEEKLY SCHEDULE          WEEK # _____          DATES _____

| ACTIVITIES | Mon | Tue | Wed | Thu | Fri | Sat | Sun |
|---|---|---|---|---|---|---|---|
| 3 Daily Meals | — | — | — | — | — | — | — |
| 3 Daily Snacks | — | — | — | — | — | — | — |
| Nutrients as Scheduled | — | — | — | — | — | — | — |
| 40 Minutes Exercise (4 Times Weekly) | — | — | — | — | — | — | — |
| Sauna | — | — | — | — | — | — | — |
| Yoga, Tai Chi, Qigong | — | — | — | — | — | — | — |
| Homework: Reading, Journaling, etc. | — | — | — | — | — | — | — |
| Food Planning, Shopping | — | — | — | — | — | — | — |
| Meal Preparation | — | — | — | — | — | — | — |
| Quality Family Relations | — | — | — | — | — | — | — |
| Quality Support Time | — | — | — | — | — | — | — |
| Quality Alone Time | — | — | — | — | — | — | — |
| Fun, Relaxation | — | — | — | — | — | — | — |

WEEKLY SCHEDULE          WEEK # _____          DATES _____

| ACTIVITIES | Mon | Tue | Wed | Thu | Fri | Sat | Sun |
|---|---|---|---|---|---|---|---|
| 3 Daily Meals | — | — | — | — | — | — | — |
| 3 Daily Snacks | — | — | — | — | — | — | — |
| Nutrients as Scheduled | — | — | — | — | — | — | — |
| 40 Minutes Exercise (4 Times Weekly) | — | — | — | — | — | — | — |
| Sauna | — | — | — | — | — | — | — |
| Yoga, Tai Chi, Qigong | — | — | — | — | — | — | — |
| Homework: Reading, Journaling, etc. | — | — | — | — | — | — | — |
| Food Planning, Shopping | — | — | — | — | — | — | — |
| Meal Preparation | — | — | — | — | — | — | — |
| Quality Family Relations | — | — | — | — | — | — | — |
| Quality Support Time | — | — | — | — | — | — | — |
| Quality Alone Time | — | — | — | — | — | — | — |
| Fun, Relaxation | — | — | — | — | — | — | — |

WEEKLY SCHEDULE  WEEK # _____  DATES _____

| ACTIVITIES | Mon | Tue | Wed | Thu | Fri | Sat | Sun |
|---|---|---|---|---|---|---|---|
| 3 Daily Meals | — | — | — | — | — | — | — |
| 3 Daily Snacks | — | — | — | — | — | — | — |
| Nutrients as Scheduled | — | — | — | — | — | — | — |
| 40 Minutes Exercise (4 Times Weekly) | — | — | — | — | — | — | — |
| Sauna | — | — | — | — | — | — | — |
| Yoga, Tai Chi, Qigong | — | — | — | — | — | — | — |
| Homework: Reading, Journaling, etc. | — | — | — | — | — | — | — |
| Food Planning, Shopping | — | — | — | — | — | — | — |
| Meal Preparation | — | — | — | — | — | — | — |
| Quality Family Relations | — | — | — | — | — | — | — |
| Quality Support Time | — | — | — | — | — | — | — |
| Quality Alone Time | — | — | — | — | — | — | — |
| Fun, Relaxation | — | — | — | — | — | — | — |

WEEKLY SCHEDULE          WEEK # _____          DATES _____

| ACTIVITIES | Mon | Tue | Wed | Thu | Fri | Sat | Sun |
|---|---|---|---|---|---|---|---|
| 3 Daily Meals | — | — | — | — | — | — | — |
| 3 Daily Snacks | — | — | — | — | — | — | — |
| Nutrients as Scheduled | — | — | — | — | — | — | — |
| 40 Minutes Exercise (4 Times Weekly) | — | — | — | — | — | — | — |
| Sauna | — | — | — | — | — | — | — |
| Yoga, Tai Chi, Qigong | — | — | — | — | — | — | — |
| Homework: Reading, Journaling, etc. | — | — | — | — | — | — | — |
| Food Planning, Shopping | — | — | — | — | — | — | — |
| Meal Preparation | — | — | — | — | — | — | — |
| Quality Family Relations | — | — | — | — | — | — | — |
| Quality Support Time | — | — | — | — | — | — | — |
| Quality Alone Time | — | — | — | — | — | — | — |
| Fun, Relaxation | — | — | — | — | — | — | — |

# END NOTES

## CHAPTER ONE
### The OLD Alcoholism Story

1 Francis Hartigan, *Bill W*, P.205-208
2 *Bill Wilson, A Second Communication to AA Physicians,* 1968. Reprinted by the Huxley Institute for Biosocial Research, 900 North Federal Highway, Boca Raton, FL, 33432
3 *"Biotype and Nutritional Status of Alcohol Dependent Medical Detoxification Inpatients Survey,"* Suka Chapel, RN, PhD, 2009
4 Research by the Laboratory of Biometry and Epidemiology, published March 23, 2009, IAAA News Release

## CHAPTER TWO
### The NEW Alcoholism Story – Reward Deficiency Syndrome

1 Research by the Laboratory of Biometry and Epidemiology, published March 23, 2009, IAAA News Release

## CHAPTER FOUR
### Depression Uncovered

1 U.S. Environmental Protection Agency, 2010
2 *Seven Weeks to Sobriety*, Joan Mathews Larson, PhD. 1997, page 244
3 *Seven Weeks to Sobriety*, Joan Mathews Larson, PhD. 1997, page 261
4 Williams and Kalita, Orthomolecular Medicine
5 J. Tintera, *"Stabilizing Homeostasis in the Recovering Alcoholic through Endocrine Therapy: Evaluation of the Hypoglycemic Factor, "* Journal of American Geriatrics 14. no. 2 (1966): p 71, 90, 92
6 *"Biotype and Nutritional Status of Alcohol Dependent Medical Detoxification Inpatients Survey,"* Suka Chapel, RN, PhD, 2009
7 *Addiction The Hidden Epidemic*, Pam Killeen, Xlibris Corporation, p.178

## CHAPTER FIVE
### Finding the Underlying Cause

1 These tests have been derived from leading experts in the field of health and wellness, including William Crook, MC, Julia Ross, MA, Joan Mathews-Larson, PhD, George Kroker, MD, and William Walsh, PhD.

## CHAPTER ELEVEN
### Food Allergies

1 *The Mood Cure* by Julia Ross, MA, p 137

## CHAPTER FIFTEEN
### Attention Deficit (Hyperactivity) Disorder

1 *Overload - Attention Deficit Disorder and the Addictive Brain* – David Miller & Kenneth Blum, PhD

## CHAPTER NINETEEN
### Biochemical Repair Simplified

1 *Mental and Elemental Nutrients*, C. Pfeiffer, New Canaan,Conn.: Keats, 1975
2 *New Hope for Incurable Diseases, E. Charaskin and W. Ringsdorf, (New York: Arco, 1971)*, pages 61-62
3 *Florida Medical Examiners Commission 2008*
4 *The Side Effects of Side Effects*, Patricia Barry, AARP.org/bulletin, September 2011
5 Joseph D. Beasley, MD and Susan Knightly, *Food for Recovery: The Complete Nutritional Companion for Recovering from Alcoholism, Drug Addiction and Eating Disorders* (New York: Crown Publishers, 1994), p. 53

## CHAPTER TWENTY SEVEN
### Nicotine Addiction

1 Mansvelder, H.D., Keath, J.R., and McGehee, D.S. *"Nicotine itself directly induces stimulation in the brain reward areas." Neuron* 33[6]:905-919, 2002
2 *A New Prescription for Addiction,* Richard I. Gracer, MD, page 246
3 From Wikipedia, the free encyclopedia
4 Lerman, C.s, et al. *"Pharmacogenetic investigation of smoking cessation treatment."* Pharmacogenetics 12(8): 627-634, 2002

## CHAPTER TWENTY EIGHT
### Body Repair

1 Contributed by Emmele Judycki, RN, BSN, Certified Quantum Touch Professional Instructor

## CHAPTER TWENTY NINE
### Self Repair

1 *Change Your Brain, Change Your Life,* Daniel G. Amen,MD
2 *Discover the Power of Meridian Tapping*, Patricia Carrington, PhD, 2008, Book Jacket

## CHAPTER THIRTY TWO
### PAWS / AD(H)D

1 *Overload –Attention Deficit Disorder and the Addictive Brain* – David Miller & Kenneth Blum, PhD

# APPENDIX A

## RECOVERY RESOURCES

### CONSULTATIONS

If you have specific questions about the information in this book or how to work this program, you can request a consultation with Dr. Suka. www.BrainworksAlcoholRecovery.com.

### MANAGED DO-IT-YOURSELF PROGRAM

If you want to pursue the Do-It-Yourself recovery program at home but are feeling overwhelmed, you can choose a Managed Program instead. This program consists of a telephone assessment with Dr. Suka who will create an amino and co-factor protocol that is individualized for your specific needs. Your supplements will be shipped directly to you. You will have an in-depth consultation on how to begin your program and on-going consultations will guide and support you throughout your recovery program. www.BrainworksAlcoholRecovery.com.

### ARISE ALCOHOL RECOVERY RESIDENTIAL
### AFTERCARE AND RELAPSE PROGRAMS

Some individuals will be able to successfully end their addiction to alcohol by following the guidelines in this book. Others may benefit from a residential program that offers individual education, guidance, and support.

Most of our residents have been through other treatment programs, or have tried AA, and have relapsed, often several times. They want something different and are highly motivated to do whatever it takes to recover.

This program stresses symptom-free recovery versus sobriety. The program uses a biochemical approach to recovery, similar to the one outlined in this book, combined with other natural modalities including a Life Skills Program. Residents live in the home with Dr. Suka and her husband, David, a recovery coach. www.AriseAlcoholRecovery.com.

### CONCIERGE RESIDENTIAL PROGRAM

Clients can decide where they want to do their residential treatment program. Dr. Suka and her husband David will bring the treatment program to the client at their home or to most any location of the client's choice in the U.S. www.AriseAlcoholRecovery.com.

# APPENDIX B

# RECOMMENDED RESOURCES

## LABORATORY TESTING
## DIRECT HEALTH

www.pyroluriatesting.com

A large variety of tests are available from Direct Health including, but not limited to, tests for pyroluria, histamine, copper and zinc. They can be ordered directly by the client, or through a healthcare provider or through Dr. Suka. Insurance may cover these tests.

## SANESCO INTERNATIONAL

http://www.sanescohealth.com

Sanesco Health offers testing for neurotransmitters and adrenal insufficiency. The tests can be ordered directly by the client, through a healthcare provider or through Dr. Suka. Insurance coverage is available.

## LIFE EXTENSION

www.lef.org

Life Extension offers many tests that are available to the public without a prescription. There is no insurance coverage for these tests.

## VITAMIN D COUNCIL

www.vitamindcouncil.com

Inexpensive and accurate Vitamin D testing.

## INSURANCE

Be aware that a diagnostic code must be attached to all insurance requests. Some people prefer to pay out-of-pocket in order to avoid having a diagnostic label attached to their medical records for life.

# APPENDIX C

## BIOCHEMICAL RESTORATION EXPERTS

JULIA ROSS, MA, MFT, author of *The Mood Cure* and *Diet Cure,* Executive Director of The Recovery Systems. 415-383-3611   www.dietcure.com

JOAN MATHEWS-LARSON, PhD, author of *Seven Weeks to Sobriety* and *Depression Free Naturally*. Director:  Health Recovery Center. 800-554-9155   www.HealthRecovery.com

HYLA CASS, MD, author of *Natural Highs, Feel Good All the Time* and *8 Weeks to Vibrant Health,*   www.cassmd.com

WILLIAM J. WALSH, PHD, author of *Nutrient Power, Heal Your Biochemistry And Heal Your Brain,* www.walshinstitute.org.

# APPENDIX D

## BIOCHEMICAL RECOVERY BOOKS

*"Why Do I Feel This Way?" Natural Relief from Moods and Depression*—Suka Chapel-Horst, RN, PhD

*Natural Highs – Feel Good All the Time* —Hyla Cass, MD & Patrick Holford

*8 Weeks to Vibrant Health* – Hyla Cass, MD & Kathleen Barnes

*Mood Cure*—Julia Ross, MA, MFT

*Diet Cure* —Julia Ross, MA, MFT

*Seven Weeks to Sobriety*—Joan Mathews Larson, PhD

*Depression Free Naturally*—Joan Mathews Larson, PhD

*Understanding your Mind, Mood, and Hormone Cycle* – Leslie Carol Botha, H. Sandra Chevalier-Batik

*Brain Longevity* – Dharma Singh Khalsa, MD

*Food & Behavior* – Barbara Reed Stitt, PhD

*Nutrient Power, Heal Your Biochemistry And Heal Your Brain*, William J. Walsh, PhD.

*The Vitamin Cure for Alcoholism* - Abram Hoffer, MD, PhD and Andrew W. Saul, PhD.

*End Your Addiction Now—The Proven Nutritional Supplement Program That Can Set You Free*—Charles Gant, MD, PhD, and Greg Lewis, PhD

*The Edge Effect* – Eric R. Braverman, MD

*Overload – Attention Deficit Disorder and the Addictive Brain* – David Miller and Kenneth Blum, PhD

*Addiction—The Hidden Epidemic*—Pam Killeen

*Food Allergy and Nutrition Revolution*—James Braly, MD

*Nutrition and Physical Degeneration*—Weston A. Price, DDS

*Change your Brain, Change your Life*—Daniel G. Amen, MD, (SPECT Brain Scan)

*Anatomy of an Epidemic* – Robert Whitaker

# APPENDIX E

## PERSONAL SUPPORT BOOKS/CDS/DVDS

### BOOKS

*Ancient Secret of the Fountain of Youth* - Peter Kelder & Bernie S. Siegel, MD

*Discover the Power of Meridian Tapping* - Patricia Carrington, PhD

*Neuro-Linguistic Programming for Dummies* - Romilla Ready, Kate Burton

*Excuses Begone* - Wayne W. Dyer, PhD

*Zero Limits* - Joe Vitale & Ihaleakala Hew Len, PhD, (Ho'oponopono)

*Limitless You* - Lee Gerdes (Brain Technologies)

*Dr. Atkins' Carbohydrate Gram Counter* - Robert C. Atkins, MD

*Prescription for Nutritional Healing* - Phyllis A. Balch, CNC

### CD'S & DVD'S

*The NEW Alcoholism Story - Reward Deficiency Syndrome, Suka Chapel-Horst, RN, PhD, CD*

*The Real Cause and Solution for Alcohol Addiction, Suka Chapel-Horst, RN, PhD, DVD*

*Say "Goodbye" to Moods and Depression, Suka Chapel-Horst, RN, PhD, DVD*

*The Tapping Solution - Nick Ortner, DVD*

*Operation Emotional Freedom – DVD www.operation-emotionalfreedom.com*

*The Shadow Effect - Debbie Ford, DVD*

*Excuses Begone - Dr. Wayne W. Dyer, CD*

*Wishes Fulfilled - Dr. Wayne W. Dyer, CD*

*Which Brain Do You Want? - Daniel G. Amen, MD (SPECT Brain Scan), DVD*

*The Secret—Law of Attraction, DVD*

# ABOUT THE AUTHOR

*"Dr. Suka"* Chapel-Horst, RN, PhD, is the author of *"Why Do I Feel This Way?" Natural Relief from Moods and Depression.* She is the founder and director of *ARISE* Alcohol Recovery, a residential aftercare and relapse program, Brainworks Alcohol Recovery offering Do-It-Yourself alcohol recovery programs, and Brainworks Recovery, an educational and consulting practice. She serves clients across the U.S.

Dr. Suka has degrees in Nursing, Business, Human Resources, Ministry, Metaphysics and is an interfaith Ordained Minister. She is also a Master Practitioner of Neuro-Linguistics and an EFT (Emotional Freedom Techniques) Practitioner.

Dr. Suka has been an RN for over 40 years, specializing in the fields of Mental Health, Criminal Justice and Drug Dependency in Minnesota, Washington, Colorado and North Carolina.

She was a national speaker and corporate trainer for 15 years, as well as President of Personal Growth Foundation, an educational organization that wrote and provided training programs to over 80,000 participants nationally.

Dr. Suka created and directed the highly successful Peers Optimal Health Program conducted in five centers in Minneapolis and St. Paul, MN. In that program over six hundred participants achieved improved health and weight loss, as well as emotional, mental and spiritual upliftment. Pre-existing medical conditions were decreased or eliminated through a combination of biochemical restoration, energy balancing and psychosocial education.

Dr. Suka has been a ski instructor, a National Ski Patrol First Aid Instructor certified in Mountain and Avalanche Rescue, First Aid Instructor and Disaster Representative for the American Red Cross and Professional Rescue Instructor of Minnesota. She has served as a Victim Advocate for the Boulder, CO Police Department and Chaplain for the Boulder County, CO Sheriff's Department. Dr. Suka was a Hospital Chaplain for Presbyterian Hospital in Denver, CO.

Dr. Suka, her husband David, and their Pomeranian, Peekaboo, travel in their motor home throughout the U.S. giving presentations and workshops.

www.AriseAlcoholRecovery.com
www.BrainworksAlcoholRecovery.com
www.BrainworksRecovery.com

Printed in Great Britain
by Amazon

11243941R00111